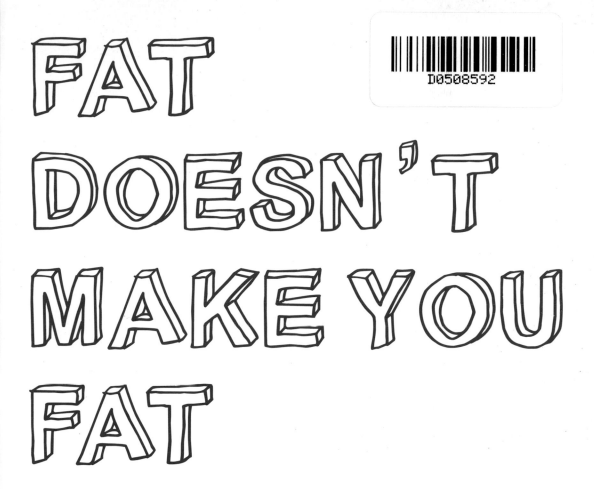

FAT DOESN'T MAKE YOU FAT

And other naked health truths

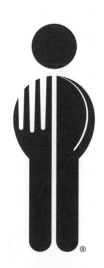

Khush Mark PhD

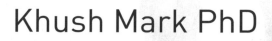

Published by Effervescent Life

Published 2008

©Khush Mark 2008

ISBN 978 0 9561298 0 2

Edited by Teresa Palmeiro

Book design by Peg Design www.pegdesign.co.uk

Illustrations by Anna Lubecka and Kierstie Masih

Printed and bound in the UK by Broglia Press

The advice given in this book is not intended to be a substitute for the advice and counsel of your personal physician. The author and publisher can not be held responsible for any loss or claim arising out of the use or misuse of the information provided or the failure to take medical advice.

To David, Indie and Jai it is because of you that this book has been possible, thank you for allowing me to hibernate away and put it together. David you have been an amazing support through it all, you are wonderful!

To my extended family and beautiful friends your feedback and encouragement has been invaluable.

To all my patients, students and lecturers you have taught me so much and continue to do so and please don't stop now.

I would also like to thank Teresa for her incredible thoroughness and detailed work. Anna and Kierstie for the illustrations and last but not at all least Mike for putting the whole book together and your positive words and energy.

Bless you all!

I dedicate this book to my parents

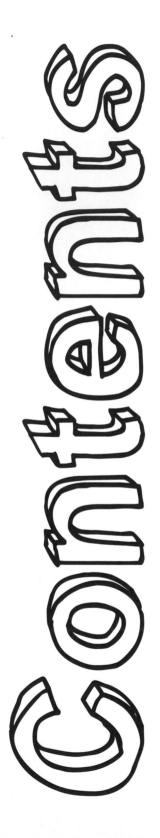

Contents

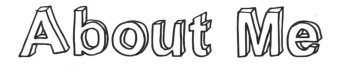

About Me

My first encounter with the wonders of the human body was when my sister, at the age of three fell over and cut her knee. All I remember was the copious amount of blood that gushed out from her wound. From this incidence onward I became fascinated with how our bodies work and resulted in me gaining a degree in Pharmacology, a Master's in Toxicology and Pathology and a PhD in cancer. Once I had completed my PhD I worked for a health clinic in London where I gained a passion to educate people on the importance of a healthy lifestyle in the prevention of disease.

Later, I went onto complete a Masters in Human Nutrition in North America and now back in the UK I run a practice in Harley Street, London. I see people from all age groups with all types of conditions, ranging from obesity, diabetes, chronic fatigue, multiple sclerosis through to cancer. I love seeing people achieve optimal health and pursue their goals in life!

My clinical experience and my clients have given me the passion and conviction to write this book and spread the news that simple, healthy eating have untold benefits for the body. So kick off those shoes and enjoy. If time is pressing right now, why not start with the Introduction and hopefully tomorrow will bring another few stolen minutes and before you know it, you will be educated into eating 'healthily', resulting in a healthier YOU.

Introduction

Have you ever thought about losing some weight, boosting your energy levels or tackling a condition that is reducing the quality of your life but have been overwhelmed by the conflicting nutritional advice?

If so then you are in for a treat. I believe many of us are being confused by the overwhelming number of diets which vary from the low fat to the alkaline diet. I am going to introduce you to a new attitude towards food and some simple basics of healthy eating. This means no calorie counting, no weighing of food and an understanding of how the body reacts to certain 'bad' foods. I hope that I will not only improve your health and well being but also clear up any confusion once and for all.

With more and more low fat foods available such as margarines, low fat yoghurts, skimmed milk, reduced fat ready made meals, more organic produce, constant research and government spending on health concerns like obesity, diabetes, high cholesterol and high blood pressure, you would think that these health issues would be on the decline. This however is not the case.

Your body is a complex being, not only is it made up of a physical body but also an incredibly powerful mind. In order to be healthy overall, you need to be physically, mentally, emotionally and spiritually healthy. Addressing one without the other is like inflating a punctured car tyre.

Some of the things you will learn include the importance of;

- eating three meals a day with a balance of protein, carbohydrate and fat
- eating 'good fats' for which your brain will be forever grateful since it is about 60% fat itself
- eating regularly throughout the day to avoid energy slumps and weight gain
- cutting out manufactured synthetic fats which are toxic and known as the 'bad' fats
- understanding that we are not only what we eat but also what we think

The information in this book is simple, there is no rocket science involved that we do not already know about in the world of nutritional medicine. If we feed our body both physically and emotionally the basic building blocks, the results are pretty astounding. Some of you may require additional nutrient support in the form of supplements or others may need to avoid certain foods due to allergies/intolerances but once we get the basics right you can move on from there.

Most frequent food and health questions

 You say that each meal should be a balance of carbohydrates, good fats and protein. Why can't I just have rice with vegetables and cashew nuts and leave out the protein? It must be healthier, as it is lower in fat and therefore calories?

It is vital to erase that 'tape' and play a new message, which is 'just because a meal is lower in calories it does not mean it is healthy, even if those calories are from wholesome organic non protein sources'. It is not about the quantity of food and so calories but about the quality! The body does not function very well (especially the stress glands called the adrenals) on meals that are not balanced with all the food groups: carbohydrates, proteins and good fats. When the adrenals are not happy, then the liver or any other organ or system for that matter, will be upset too.

Q If I eat protein and fat as you suggest won't my cholesterol levels go up?

A It is a myth that fat increases cholesterol because our cholesterol levels are regulated by the liver. But most importantly and this is something that very few people know, is that cholesterol is a healing agent. If you implement the Naked Truth lifestyle cholesterol levels will not increase unless you have an injury or any other particular stress where cholesterol is used by the body to heal the 'damage'.

Dietary factors that increase cholesterol are the basic stimulants such as white refined carbohydrates (bread, pasta etc), alcohol, caffeine, hydrogenated fats, the so-called 'artificial' foods, artificial sweeteners and drugs. In other words foods that do not exist in nature and man made synthetic chemicals. Why? Because they create damage within the body and cholesterol is then produced to heal and repair this damage.

Q But I have been advised to stay away from fat especially saturated due to my high cholesterol levels?

Sure, but read the response to the question above. It is important to remember that cholesterol is a healing agent and not 'harmful' as it has been made out to be. The question we need to ask is why is my cholesterol high? What damage is there in my body that it is trying to heal? Why do I need to heal? Is it because I am drinking coffee regularly or unhappy at work?

Won't I gain weight eating all these food groups in every meal?

No, this is not possible. It is all about regulating blood sugar balance. If you can maintain a healthy blood sugar balance there is no excess sugar to store as fat. In addition, once your blood sugar level is stable your body does not crave more food than it needs so you may well find that you lose weight.

I feel really 'heavy' if I combine protein with whole grains (the carbohydrate) such as brown rice, so what can I do?

In my experience quite a few people have digestive imbalances (look out for Susan's husband, Steve) the symptoms can vary from bloating, excess flatulence, burping, constipation, acid reflux and abdominal pain. In such cases I would recommend having salads and vegetables as your sources of carbohydrates with protein and fat until the digestive system is balanced. The digestive system usually takes time to adapt when changing from a diet that is full of unhealthy foods and synthetic chemicals.

So if it is not about the quantity but about the quality of food can I eat twice as much?

In my clinical experience it is rare that individuals eat more when they follow the Naked Truth lifestyle. Once the blood sugar is on an 'even keel' the hunger actually reduces. If after following this lifestyle for 4 weeks you are still hungry within 2 hours of eating your balanced meal then other metabolic imbalances need to be analysed.

Can I have breakfast once I get to work?

This is not recommended. In order to maintain or achieve great health, breakfast should be eaten within 30-40 minutes of waking up.

Is it true that table salt is unhealthy but there are other salts that are important for good health?

If we look back at the history of table salt, you will discover primarily that regular table salt is sodium chloride and sodium chloride was originally used for the manufacture of various materials including PVC! I would suggest avoiding regular refined salt such as standard table salt and switching to the more non refined salt like the Himalayan salt or the Celtic sea salt which contains a whole host of minerals that are vital for good health. Such unrefined salt is essential for good health.

Do I have to be 'good' all the time or am I allowed 'treats'?

The 80:20 rule is pretty important. By this I mean try and stick with eating healthily 80% of the time with 20% 'treat' time. But just as important as eating healthily is taking care of your emotional well being. What will you gain if you are eating healthily but are dissatisfied, stressed, unhappy in your relationship etc?

I have an under active thyroid; will the Naked Truth lifestyle help me?

This programme is for anyone who wants to get healthy whether they have a diagnosed condition or not, so yes it will help you. From experience I have found that in most cases the underlying cause of an under active thyroid is 'over-worked' stress glands, the adrenals. It is quite common for adrenal stress to be confused with low thyroid activity.

There are differing views on juicing, what is your view and why?

I am not an avid believer in juicing as I believe that it is more wholesome to eat the whole vegetable and/or fruit in its entirety. Fruit juicing is not recommended due to the negative impact on blood sugar levels. Green vegetable juicing can be beneficial for those people who have been diagnosed with specific conditions such as cancer but it is always ideal to obtain nutrients from the whole food. The green vegetables do not create such blood sugar stress whereas fruit juices can. Not only that but juicing removes the fibre from these fruits which further increases the blood sugar boosting properties of the fruit. The favourite apple and carrot juice with ginger for breakfast can create an unhealthy rise in blood sugar levels that throws the body out of balance, which can lead to you feeling off balance for the rest of the day. If juicing vegetables I would still encourage you to eat the pulp too!

I have an orange juice or apple juice every morning with my breakfast to boost my nutrient levels, is there any other drink that you would also recommend?

Firstly it is great that you are thinking of boosting your nutrient levels but doing this by having a fruit juice is doing you more harm than good. I always suggest a herbal tea. My concern about fruit juices is their harsh impact on blood sugar levels. Also in one glass of apple juice (about 240 millilitres) you get all the fruit sugar from 1587 grammes of apples without the fibre! This is pretty 'heavy going' on the body not to mention that for the rest of the day your body will be craving more sugar.

Q Is fructose (also known as fruit sugar) a healthier option instead of standard sugar?

 A No. At one time it was believed that because fructose does not have an impact on insulin levels it was therefore a healthy alternative to sugar. So it has been used to sweeten foods such as cereals, ready made meals, beverages, breads, biscuits etc However, fructose can only be metabolised by the liver and once consumed goes straight to the liver, increasing the liver's 'work load'. Here the fructose is converted indirectly to fat which can have a negative impact on the cardiovascular system such as the heart, blood pressure etc. Fructose can also create insulin resistance which can result in various health problems from obesity through to diabetes.

Q I have been recommended an alkalinising diet, so I am avoiding meat and taking an alkalinising powder daily, can I still implement the Naked Truth lifestyle?

A Anyone can implement the Naked Truth lifestyle whether they are trying to alkalinise their system or not. However, one question you have to ask yourself is 'why are you acidic in the first place?' In general the answer to this is that when our detox organs, such as the liver, kidneys, lungs, skin and bowels are not functioning optimally then toxins build up in our body which create the acidity. So cutting out meat and taking an alkalinising powder is not actually addressing the 'cause' of the acidity. This is indicated by the very fact that when you stop taking the alkalinising powder and re-introduce meat the system will become acidic again. If you implement the Naked Truth lifestyle alongside some of the organ support (provided in the Getting Going chapter) then the acidity should no longer be an issue.

History to our current eating habits

Thousands of years ago humans lived a very different lifestyle. Food was a different 'breed' in that it was natural and stresses mainly involved being chased by a beast out in the wild. Although they had to deal with diseases that we do not encounter today such as plagues, life was at a much slower pace than in the 21st century.

Today, we live fast-paced, sedentary lives and survive on stimulants such as caffeine, chocolate, cakes, biscuits, alcohol, face a multitude of stresses at work and end the day by crashing out on the sofa in front of the hypnotising television screen. Our frenetic lifestyle has led to the manufacture of convenience foods which include highly damaging ingredients such as glucose-fructose syrup, partially hydrogenated fats, 'deadly' foods such as sugar and nerve deadening ingredients such as colourings and preservatives. And to top all of that we face 'new' diseases such as obesity, diabetes, Alzheimer's, cancer (just to name a few) which are impacting our quality of life.

Our frenetic lifestyle has led to the manufacture of convenience foods

Farming methods have also changed which includes the use of pesticides and the once fertile soil is now being depleted of vital nutrients. Dare I say, even 'raw organic milk' was available more readily, now it is frowned upon or treated like it is 'poisonous' and full of disease 'causing' microbes.

Many of us regularly rush off to work without breakfast. We don't worry too much about that as we usually pick up a coffee with a low fat muffin on the way to the office. Some of us manage to eat lunch whereas other's just grab another stimulant, be it a cake, chocolate bar or another coffee. Well, why not, it keeps you going for an extra few minutes? Then in the afternoon the energy slump hits and another stimulant is consumed which doesn't even stimulate the taste buds, it just goes straight down the gullet...roll on 'home time'.

in the afternoon the energy slump hits and another stimulant is consumed

As we keep feeding our bodies stimulants such as coffee and sugar (in the muffin, chocolate, cake etc) our blood sugar levels keep spiking. When the sugar is too high in the blood it can start to create all sorts of internal chaos resulting in weight gain, heart disease, low energy, poor concentration, diabetes and so on.

On the way home, everyone seems rather tired but just manage to make the journey home to collapse on the sofa. Some of us may be so tired that we even get a few winks on the train or bus home, how convenient, but maybe not for the passenger on the next seat. The tiredness we are feeling is because the body is working hard to bring down the excess sugar in our system in order to prevent long-term ill health. However, the sugar level then plummets too low and manifests itself as tiredness, sleepiness, irritability, increased susceptibility to infections, further cravings for stimulants like coffee, sugar and so on.

In through the front door, you may be greeting your children or coming back home after picking them up from a nursery or childminder, or you may be going home to your flatmate or partner with no children in tow and then, there are some of us going home to our own little 'pad' in 'peace'.

Whatever the house dynamics you can easily achieve good vibrant health by physically and emotionally feeding the body with the basic building blocks some of which include:

- having three square meals a day with all three food groups (carbohydrate, protein and fat) and not forgetting to snack
- drinking water throughout the day
- cutting out artificial sweeteners which means avoiding diet drinks and low fat desserts
- ensuring you are sleeping well
- having a positive outlook on life

So let me introduce you to the three food groups...

Cholestrol is a healing agent. Chlestrol levels are regulated by LIVER. factors that increase cholestrol are bacteria + invlents —

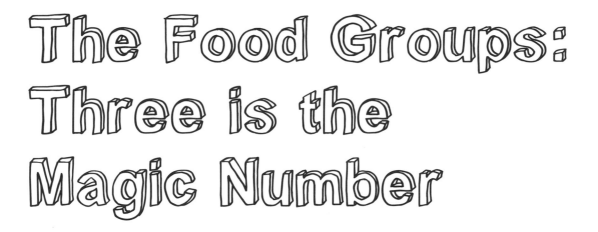

The Food Groups: Three is the Magic Number

In order to establish healthy eating I would like to introduce you to the basic three food groups. Each basic food group has a vital role in building and maintaining great health.

Over the past several decades we have seen the introduction of 'synthetic' man made 'foods', such as refined carbohydrates, hydrogenated fats, artificial sweeteners and so on. Their introduction has lead to the increase in disease from obesity through to cancer. These products strictly do not belong to any of the basic food groups although they tend to be categorised as such. The three basic food groups include carbohydrates, proteins and fats. Each meal must consist of all three food groups, carbohydrates, proteins and fats.

Group 1: Carbohydrates

Most of us love carbohydrates and generally want more. When asked to name carbohydrates we come up with: potatoes, rice, bread and pasta BUT **do not forget salads, vegetables, fruits and whole grains.**

The body breaks carbohydrates down to basic sugar units which mainly provide energy. Most of us have probably heard of 'carbohydrate loading' that goes on before a marathon, be it a tri-athalon or a mini-marathon, which is all to provide energy for the fuel zapping event.

Breads and pasta (also known as the pre-baked grains) are really what are called high glycaemic index (GI) foods. In other words they flood the blood with sugar (which comes from these high GI carbohydrate foods) very quickly. High blood sugar can injure blood vessels that serve a number of key organs in the body such as the eyes, heart and kidneys but it can also slow down the healing process, immune system and disrupt the metabolism.

When sugar floods into the blood stream 'all hell breaks loose'. The pancreas which is an organ in the body responsible for lowering the blood sugar levels panics and over reacts causing the sugar in the blood to come crashing down. The adrenals (which basically act as survival glands that boost our energy levels when we are being threatened and need to fight or run) react to the low blood sugar levels and believe that you are just about to be eaten alive by a wild savage beast. When the adrenals are triggered in this manner their response is to increase the level of sugar in the blood stream. So we have a vicious cycle where the pancreas and adrenals are made to work over time. The strain on these internal organs constantly dealing with unhealthy levels of sugar in the blood lead to a plethora of symptoms from weight gain through to chronic fatigue.

When sugar floods into the blood stream 'all hell breaks loose'

This internal drama is caused by pre-baked or so-called high GI carbohydrates but sadly for the chocolate addicts, pastry lovers or muffin buffins among us these 'junk' foods create exactly the same chaos within the body. Such 'foods' are broken down into sugar very rapidly creating this vicious cycle. To achieve great health we must feed our body so that we avoid these blood sugar extremes.

Group 2: Proteins

Protein foods tend to be low on the list for most folk, especially if we are following a low fat diet. These foods include fish, meat (both lean and not-so-lean meat), dairy, lentils, beans, pulses and fermented soya products such as tempeh, tofu, nato etc. Dairy in my book really refers to cheese (not milk) and the lentils, beans and pulses include kidney beans, chick peas, haricot beans and so on.

Proteins are broken down by our amazing digestive system into amino acids. Such amino acids are involved in a multitude of functions in the body, one of them being to maintain a healthy immune system which fights off diseases. Others include the building of brain chemicals such as serotonin which is our 'happy chemical'. These brain chemicals keep our emotional balance in check.

Amino acids can also be found in supplement form. For example an amino acid called glutamine can be and has been used to feed the starving brain. By feeding the brain this amino acid the hunger pangs die down for a while. In other words glutamine in supplement form has an appetite suppressant type role, but short cuts like this only create long-term health problems because the body still needs nourishing in order to heal and repair and avoid ill health as well as gain great health.

Here are a few other useful roles of protein:

- healthy skin
- boosts the metabolism
- helps with healing damage
- hormonal balance
- balancing mood
- cleansing of the body

Group 3: Fats

Most people shudder at the thought of fats and I am not surprised because we are constantly being informed that fats are bad for us. However, the information we are being given is confused and in some respects incorrect. Although bad fats do exist and we do need to avoid them because they contribute to conditions such as heart disease, there are various fats that are not only good fats but are vital for good health.

good fats come from natural sources

Bad Fats

Put simply bad fats are called hydrogenated fats and are 'synthetic' manufactured fats and the good fats come from natural sources, for example olive oil, sesame seed oil, butter etc. As a nation we have been encouraged to switch from butter (a good fat) to margarines or 'spreadable' oils which are the bad fats that are slowly poisoning our bodies.

Hydrogenated fats are fats that have been through the hydrogenation process. This is where vegetable oil is reacted under pressure with hydrogen gas at 250 - 400°F for several hours in the presence of a catalyst such as nickel or platinum. This artificial process converts liquid fats into solids such as margarine.

Before the theory that 'eating foods with saturated fat causes heart disease' most of us were happy eating butter and saturated fats and using lard etc. But once saturated fats were given a bad name and blamed for a host of health problems, hydrogenated fats became the 'new trend'. Vegetable oils became the healthy option to butter and saturated fats. But there was one problem, how were we supposed to spread them on our food? Well this is where hydrogenation comes in. It is a process to solidify oil so that it can be made to resemble real foods such as butter but also imparts 'desirable' features such as spreadability, texture and increased shelf life to naturally liquid vegetable oils.

Manufacturers, started to use hydrogenated oils as they extend the shelf life of food (but not yours!). Do you ever wonder how a cake or a packet of biscuits can last for months before being opened? And don't be fooled by food labels that say "made from partially-hydrogenated fat". This is also known as a trans fat and is worse than totally hydrogenated fat. As a basic rule keep well away from any foods or oils that contain hydrogenated fats or that have been hydrogenated in any shape or form. This includes some breads, ready made low fat meals, pastries, low fat muffins, cakes, biscuits etc. Always check the food label.

Do you ever wonder how a cake or a packet of biscuits can last for months before being opened?

A result of the trend to reduce saturated fats has been the manufacture of so-called fat free or low fat foods. What we are not told, however, is that in order to replace the flavour that is lost from removing the fat, these foods tend to be rich in sugar, sometimes even containing twice as much sugar than the original 'full fat version'. One of the vital roles of fat is satiation, without fat in our meals we do not feel satiated and therefore we can continue to eat beyond our body's needs. These low fat or fat-free foods may sound healthy but these foods are responsible for the expanding girth in the UK as well as other illnesses including heart disease.

There is a slow change taking place in the food world and trans fats are now generally recognised as being unhealthy. Even the Food Standards Agency in the UK has taken the step of asking for better labelling on food products and New York is the first large city in the US to limit the use of trans fats in restaurants. On July 1 2007, restaurants were barred from frying and spreading fats containing artificial trans fats above 0.5 g per serving. By July 1, 2008 they had to meet the same target for all of their foods.

I mention hydrogenated fats as part of the fat food group only as it is widely available, but in all honesty it is not a fat but a toxin. If we looked at 'true' fats and that is those fats

Fat does not make you fat – it is a myth

that do not include hydrogenated fats then it is true to say that Fat does not make you fat – it is a myth.

Cholesterol: friend or foe?

There is also the belief that eating foods containing cholesterol and/or saturated fat will increase the level of cholesterol in your blood which will be 'dumped' in artery walls causing them to narrow. This narrowing will block the nutrient supply to various organs in the body and can cause heart disease, heart attack or stroke (depending upon where this 'narrowing' takes place), just to name the popular few. This theory is called the 'diet-heart hypothesis' and was first discovered by Ancel Keys in 1953. (Keys, A,. Atherosclerosis: A problem in newer public health. Journal of Mount Sinai Hospital 20, 118-139 1953). In essence this theory suggests that by avoiding these fats we can prevent developing heart disease.

Well, prepare yourself for the next vital piece of information, as you really should not be leaving home without it. This 'diet-heart hypothesis' has many loopholes. For some reason cholesterol has received the guilty verdict, when it is actually a healing agent. A well respected journal called the Lancet in 1960 (Chareters AD & Arya BP. Incidence of Ischaemic heart disease among Indians in Kenya. The Lancet 1, p288-289, 1960) published observations on the dietary habits and health of two groups of Indian emigrants in Kenya. The non-Muslim Indians from Gujarat lived on a lacto-vegetarian diet (no meat, fish or eggs) while the Muslim Indians from the Punjab ate meat and eggs and consumed at least twice as much milk as their Gujarati fellows BUT most interestingly did not use vegetable oil! So the non-Muslim Indians were basically 'following' the low fat diet and the Muslim Indians were living on what we consider a high fat diet. Interestingly, the mortality rate from heart disease is EQUAL in both populations.

There are many other studies that seem to have been ignored by health professionals and the food industry, probably because they did not fit the 'diet-heart hypothesis' which gathered support and directed the focus of the food industry for years afterwards onto low fat foods. If the important decision-makers had taken into consideration these studies like the study on the Indian emigrants in Kenya then who knows what different advice we would have been given over the past 50 years. It would have also changed which drugs pharmaceuticals would have developed so not the cholesterol lowering drugs.

Unfortunately, the Western world has been convinced by the low fat and cholesterol lowering theory that now bad fats (hydrogenated fats, trans fats and partially hydrogenated fats) are part and parcel of our everyday food and no one has ever looked back – hard to believe but true. How many of us are advised to AVOID eggs, red meat, butter, cream, full fat cheese and ENCOURAGED to switch to 'low fat' foods that actually contain more sugar, additives and preservatives? I think this is a very important point that schools need to address, as kids are being encouraged to follow a low fat, low salt diet (I am referring to standard table salt here). The standard table salt I can understand but fat I can not. After all, the brain consists of nearly 60% fat. If we did not eat these good fats how would our brain function? Not very well I hasten to add.

Fat has very important functions in the body which include:

- **energy**
- **satiation**
- **insulation and protection of our vital organs from injury**
- **bone health: prevention of osteoporosis as well as prevention of conditions like multiple sclerosis**
- **smooth running of the internal workings of the body**
- **manufacture of the sex hormones responsible for fertility, sex drive, hair growth and lots more**
- **source of the so-called omega fats which are also essential for internal smooth running of the body**

Every other cell in the body except the brain cells have the ability to manufacture cholesterol. The liver regulates cholesterol levels and generously provides the brain with some too. A whole host of hormones including the sexy ones are made from cholesterol. If cholesterol was not required then why would the body even bother making it? In fact, without cholesterol, you would die in a matter of days if not within hours, which explains why it is difficult to reduce cholesterol through dieting alone. Cholesterol is so incredibly important that the body will make more (see later on cholesterol) when less is ingested!

Good fats
Foods that are goods fats include:

- butter
- ghee (also known as clarified butter)
- oils (olive, flax, sunflower, walnut, hemp)
- nuts (almonds, cashews, Brazil nuts, macadamia etc)
- seeds (pumpkin, sesame, flax, sunflower)

This food group has many essential roles in the body, one of the main ones being smooth running of the internal body.

When or if cooking with fat, I would suggest using butter, coconut, ghee, or palm oil. These are saturated fats and are safe when heated (heat-stable). When cooking with oils such as sunflower oil rancid fats are created which are toxic to the body. Such oils are not heat stable, if anything they are damaged by heating. Good quality oils should come in black or opaque containers and be stored in a cool place. This indicates that they will not become rancid. They should also be cold pressed and unrefined without the use of any harmful solvents. So purchasing sunflower oil or any other oil in plastic bottles that are stored at room temperature such as we see on row upon row in the supermarket is truly a recipe for ill health.

cooking with oils such as sunflower oil rancid fats are created which are toxic to the body

Just to reiterate, natural fats that come from natural foods are good. Fats that have been treated chemically are bad. These are normally found in cakes, biscuits, some ready made burgers, ready made meals, margarines and so on. The list is pretty endless but I would suggest to always read the label. You will be surprised to see how widespread the use of these bad fats is. So start to love the good old wholesome fats and avoid the synthetic man made harmful fats.

Carbs = Rice, Pots, Pasta, Salad, Fruit, Veg, WholeGrain
⤷ energy
Pre-baked grains (breads & pasta) = high glycaemic index
                                          (GI) foods

= flood body with sugar

Proteins Fish, Meat, Dairy, Lentils, Beans, Pulses, Tofu, Soya.
⤷ Amino Acids → Maintenance + Serotonin

Fats

Bad = trans fats. = hydrogenated fats, change liquid fats to
            to solids — Margarine. = T O X I N

Cholesterol

Water: Liquid Food

As well as the three food groups equally important is good quality water. We are made up between 75-80% water and this liquid is of vital importance.

Without it our various bodily functions (mainly the so-called biochemical reactions) shut down and our bodies become a waste dumping site.

Water intake has reduced dramatically since the introduction of 'fizzy' drinks which are full of sugar and do more harm than good. Drinks that contain sugar compared with pure water actually make us even thirstier because not only are they absorbed more slowly due to the sugar but they also require water to breakdown the sugars! Without water we cannot function as our body's chemical reactions would eventually come to a halt. We need to stay hydrated with water because:

- we function better
- we concentrate better
- we don't feel hunger so much
- our complexion improves
- our bodies are able to clear out toxins
- our joints are lubricated
- our lungs function better

Fruit juices, even fruit 'smoothies' have started to replace our water intake, but these drinks contain concentrated amounts of sugar albeit fruit sugar. Fruit sugar still has the same negative blood sugar impact as does eating a carbohydrate on its own.

Our body's thirst reaction is a 'bit delayed'. In other words by the time we are thirsty we should have drunk water at least 2 hours previously! This is because 2% of body weight as water may be lost before thirst occurs. So do not wait to get thirsty before drinking water. As we mature our thirst mechanism declines, so drinking water throughout the day is very important. The bulk of water should be drunk in between meals. If one drinks too much water with meals (which is more than about 250mls) then the digestive juices get diluted and this has the impact of slowing down the digestive process, which can result in bloating, feeling 'sleepy' after meals, indigestion, excessive belching and even tiredness.

Depending on how much water is lost by the body it has differing impacts:

- **Loss of 3% of body weight as water results in decreased muscle strength**
- **Loss of 5% results in apathy and emotional instability**
- **Loss of 7% causes headache and increased body temperature**
- **Loss of 9% causes confusion**
- **Loss of 11% causes delirium**
- **Loss of 20% is usually fatal**

Drink good quality water. There are various water filtration systems and the ones that have been found to filter out more of the 'toxins' (such as metals like lead, bacteria, chemicals) are the reverse osmosis filters.

Ideally, I would recommend a glass of water on waking which replenishes the water that has been utilised overnight in healing and repairing the body. It is usually recommended that we drink between one to two litres of water per day. I would further add to this and say that if you are drinking water throughout the day and your urine colour is yellow any time of the day then you need to drink more (unless you have a pre-diagnosed kidney condition). If your urine colour is clear then you are drinking enough.

All food groups should be organic hence free from pesticides, genetic modification and other possible toxins. Water although not organic should be purified with a good quality water filter.

So there we have it, the basic three food groups; carbohydrates, proteins, fats and the magic liquid called water. Now, what we do with these food groups can promote or hinder good health.

Let's move on...

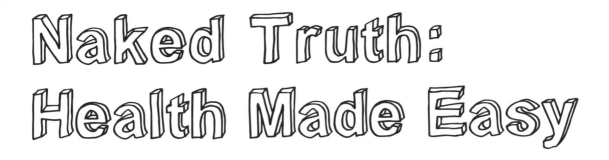

Naked Truth: Health Made Easy

EVERY meal should include ALL three food groups if you want to eat healthily and enjoy great health. That's the carbohydrates, proteins and fats and water throughout the day.

It is as easy as that, no fuss and no complicated foods with ingredients that we can't even pronounce. If you are keen on super foods and sprouting etc then by all means introduce these but most of us want a simple and healthy lifestyle. In this section I will give examples of how easily you can create healthy meals as well as examples of what is not healthy.

Healthy breakfast
Breakfast one: muesli with nuts and seeds and yoghurt with some oat milk

A bowl of muesli (sugar free) with some nuts and seeds and some natural organic whole fat yoghurt with maybe a drizzle of oat milk is healthy. Let's analyse this a bit more by looking at the protein, fat and carbohydrate components of this breakfast.

Breakdown...
- Carbohydrate: muesli, oat milk
- Protein: yoghurt
- Fat: nuts and seeds

Let's have a look at another breakfast...

Breakfast two: Scrambled eggs on rye bread toast with butter and some grilled tomatoes

Breakdown...
• Carbohydrate: rye bread and grilled tomatoes (for those who may crave ketchup which is full of sugar)
• Protein: scrambled eggs
• Fat: butter

These meals are healthy because they are balanced with all three food groups. To implement the water you can have some peppermint tea or any other caffeine free herbal tea. Always have breakfast within 30-40 minutes of waking up otherwise the body (especially the adrenal glands) can get pretty unhappy (more details later). **What is NOT a healthy option...**

Unhealthy breakfast
Breakfast one: A bowl of cereal and skimmed milk

Breakdown....
• **Carbohydrate: cereal (sweetened with glucose-fructose syrup)**
• **Protein: questionable**
• **Fat: no fat in this breakfast as the fat that could have come from the milk has been removed.**

The 'nasties' in the above breakfast are:

• **Skimmed milk**
• **Glucose-fructose syrup**
• **No protein (yes this is nasty)**

Skimmed milk is not a 'food' in my book. Milk comes with fat. It is in the fat that the fat soluble vitamins (vitamins, A, D, E and K) are found. Reducing these vital vitamins can lead to fibromyalgia (all over non specific muscle pain), multiple sclerosis and more.

it is in the fat that the fat soluble vitamins are found

If you are not sure as to whether a food is healthy or not, it is always worth asking the question 'is this food natural?'

Breakfast two: wholemeal toast with margarine and jam

Breakdown...
- **Carbohydrate: toast, jam (all high GI, the bread may also contain trans fats)**
- **Protein: none**
- **Fat: margarine if hydrogenated is a bad fat**

The 'nasties' in the above breakfast are:

- **Toast and jam and trans fats**
- **Margarine**
- **No protein (yes this is nasty)**

You have to be careful with bread, always try and read the label and watch out for sugar, trans fats, preservatives. Same with the jam, which has a huge amount of sugar in but there are brands of jam that do not add sugar. Without the protein the above meal would flood the blood with sugar and start the crazy sugar roller-coaster effect.

Lunch
In Britain, lunch tends to be a sandwich. How this nation goes through so much wheat is explained mainly by our lunch menu and typical breakfasts of toast. Let's look at some healthy lunch menus (keeping the wheat issue in mind), as well as the three food groups.

Healthy lunch

Lunch one: tuna with rocket salad, pine nuts with olive oil and lemon juice as dressing

Breakdown...
- Carbohydrate: salad
- Protein: tuna
- Fat: olive oil and pine nuts

Lunch two: brown rice, with broccoli, carrots, ginger and cashews with chicken

- Carbohydrate: brown rice and vegetables
- Protein: chicken
- Fat: cashew nuts

So include ALL three food groups in each meal with a glass of water (see the Naked Truth lifestyle weekly menu chapter for more ideas for meals).

If you are a vegetarian or vegan then opt for a vegetarian/vegan source of protein but do not omit it. Vegans would highly benefit from eating plenty of pulses, beans and fermented soya foods (not the soya protein isolate stuff which is just noxious!).

Unhealthy lunch

Lunch one: wholemeal sandwich with ham, cheese and tomato and margarine

Breakdown...
- Carbohydrate: wholemeal bread, tomato
- Protein: ham and cheese
- Fat: margarine

The 'nasties' in the above lunch are:

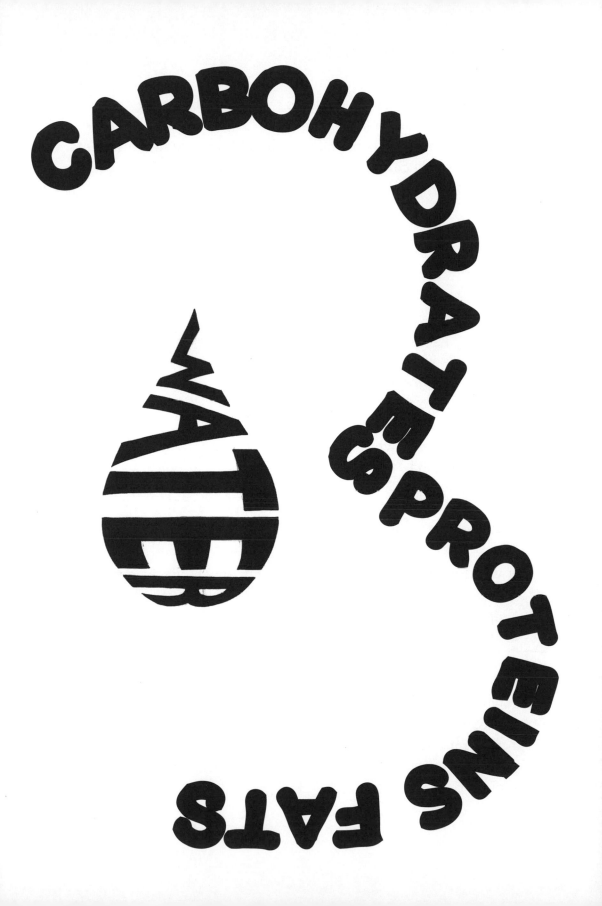

- Wholemeal bread if it contains trans fats or stimulants such as sugar – so check the label
- Margarine – as it is usually a product that contains trans fats
- Ham usually contains preservatives, sugar and high levels of salt

Always read the label as specific breads will contain the above mentioned ingredients and watch out for the processed meats that tend to be high in salt, preservatives and even sugar. Your body would have to do a lot of 'cleaning up' to try and eliminate the synthetic chemicals.

Lunch two: white pasta with mayonnaise and tuna, corn, red peppers and green salad

Breakdown...
- Carbohydrate: white pasta, corn, red peppers, green salad
- Protein: tuna
- Fat: mayonnaise

The 'nasties' in the above lunch are:

- White pasta – a refined carbohydrate which breaks down very quickly into sugar in the blood stream causing internal organs to work overtime
- Mayonnaise – because many brands contain trans fats

The above meal may seem healthy at first but when it is broken down you begin to see the 'hidden' nasties. The white pasta is a refined carbohydrate and therefore has a high sugar releasing impact into the blood stream. Most brands of mayonnaise tend to contain trans fats.

Healthy dinner

Dinner one: lamb moussaka with a salad with olive oil dressing

Breakdown...
- Carbohydrate: salad
- Protein: lamb
- Fat: olive oil

Dinner two: salmon with sautéed vegetables and partially boiled potatoes with butter

Breakdown...
- Carbohydrate: sautéed vegetables and potatoes
- Protein: salmon
- Fat: butter

Unhealthy dinner

Dinner one: wholemeal pasta with vegetables and tomato sauce

Breakdown...
- Carbohydrate: wholemeal pasta, vegetables and tomato sauce
- Protein: none
- Fat: palm oil used in cooking

The problem with this meal is that the protein is missing and the carbohydrate from the pasta will flood the blood with sugar.

Dinner two: jacket potato with some cheese and beans and butter

Breakdown....
- Carbohydrate: jacket potato
- Protein: cheese and baked beans
- Fat: butter

Nutrition Facts

Serv. Size 1 cup
Servings About 2

Calories Don't Count

Amount/Serving	%DV	Amount/Serving	%DV
Trans Fats	%	MSG	%
Hydrogenated Fats	%	Aspartame	%
Glucose-Fructose Syrup		Sugars	%
	%		

Unhealthy Ingredients

Glutamic Acid, Trans Fats, Partially Hydrogenated Oils, E678, Glucose-Fructose Syrup, Titanium, Lactic Acid, E108, Skimmed Milk Powder, E11_, Invert S___ _yrup, MSG, E12_, Sugar, ___O, Aspartam_, Sulphu___ ___ide, E450, E4__, Colou___ __480, E442, __, E671, _ ___Dioxide, E4__, Vegetab___ ___Oil, E475, __, E143, E4__ __Salt, Fa___, Reduce_ __Cocoa, E__, ___ro__ __Glucose__, ___Corn__

The 'nasties' in the dinner are the jacket potato and the beans. Potatoes that are cooked to such a degree have sugar spiking properties which can leave you feeling sleepy and tired afterwards. Generally baked beans from a can contain high levels of sugar. Look for a brand that does not contain sugar which do exist.

These are man made 'synthetic foods' which deplete nutrients

'FOODS' to avoid

I put the word 'foods' in inverted commas because these are not foods in the real sense of the word. These are man made 'synthetic foods' which deplete nutrients and in my line of work they are called nutrient robbers. These include:

- white flour products: bread, cakes, biscuits, muffins, bagels, croissants etc
- fried foods: chips, crisps, chicken nuggets, 'fry ups'
- fizzy drinks and fruit juices: especially juices from concentrates and cordials with colourings and preservatives
- confectionery: chocolate, sweets, ice creams
- unfermented soya products

Avoid foods and drinks that contain:

- additives: found in ready made meals and many of the above. These tend to start with the capital letter 'E' such as E102, E211 etc
- caffeine as found in cola drinks, coffee, certain energy-boosting beverages
- sugar (also disguised as saccharin , maltodextrin, dextrose, fructose)
- artificial sweeteners that contain aspartame, such as splenda and nutrasweet
- hydrogenated fats and trans fats

Sugar in general can be disguised in various forms and so it is beneficial to read labels and look out for these hidden sugars. They can be labelled as follows: barley malt, beet sugar, brown sugar, cane juice, cane sugar, caramel, date sugar, dextran, dextrose, fructose, fruit juice concentrate, glucose, glucose solids, golden syrup, maltodextrin, maltose, molasses, sorghum syrup, sucrose, sugar, yellow sugar. If you read the label and are not sure of any of the ingredients, go home and check it out on the internet before purchasing.

When shopping in your local supermarket you want to spend most of your money in the outside food aisles. As soon as you start to move towards the inner aisles, you will be looking at foods designed to have long shelf lives and these foods contain not only sugar but also other unwanted unhealthy preservatives.

spend most of your money in the outside food aisles

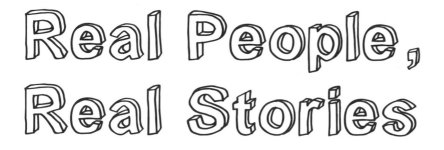

Real People, Real Stories

The cases are examples of the different types of lifestyles that we all lead whether we are the busy single mum or the young couple living together.

They all have something in common and that is they believe that eating low fat meals is healthy, that coffee is fine as long it has no sugar and suppressing emotions is 'life'. Well these are all perfect ingredients for ill health.

Until now I have been focusing on feeding the physical body, however we are complex beings, not only made up of a physical body but also an incredibly powerful mind. In order to be healthy overall, you need to be physically, mentally, emotionally and spiritually healthy. Addressing one without the other is like filling a punctured tyre with air.

No matter what our age or situation we face stress every day. It is important to be aware that stress is not necessarily the heart pumping, pulsating, perspiring experience that it's believed to be. If anything stress is basically 'the non-specific response of the body to any demand' as defined by Hans Seyle, MD, PhD who originated the concept of physiological stress. In other words a wide variety of things such as eating foods that flood the blood with sugar, watching a horror movie, doing excessive sports, being in an unhappy job can all be stressful on the body.

I am going to introduce you to some individuals who live life with daily stresses so you get the 'feel' of what stressors we can face daily in relation to our physical and emotional well being.

Although based on real cases the names of these people have been changed due to obvious reasons.

Single busy individual...Alan

Gets home and grabs a beer with some nibbles whilst heating up a ready made meal in the oven. It's a good brand and low fat. However, low fat usually indicates the presence of hydrogenated fats. As he sits down to unwind, his friend calls to see whether he wants to go out for a drink. Alan declines, as he has a work project to finish for the morning. He ends up eating his food in front of his computer and drinking three bottles of beer through the evening. Towards nine pm he starts to fall asleep at the computer and he makes himself a coffee to stay 'awake'.

the caffeine then stimulates his adrenals, the stress glands which suddenly flood the blood with sugar again

The beer has flooded his blood with sugar which triggers the vicious cycle as described earlier where the pancreas over reacts to all the sugar in the blood by mopping it all up leaving Alan feeling sleepy. By having a coffee, the caffeine then stimulates his adrenals, the stress glands which suddenly flood the blood with sugar again.

Alan is also stressed as he fears not getting a promotion. He feels his promotion will be determined by the success of this project and he cannot afford to do a 'second-rate' job. There are enough people at work waiting for promotions and this is the company's biggest financial project to date and hopefully a step up the next rung of the corporate ladder.

The body is not only fed nutritionally but also emotionally.

Exhausted mum...Susan

Susan has spent most of the day out in the park with other mums and their children and it is nearly dinner time. She chats to her children whilst gathering together the ingredients for the evening meal. Today it is a healthy dinner as yesterday was one of those 'throw it in the oven pizza' jobs. They have had too many quick meals this week. She gives the children a box of biscuits to keep them 'quiet' and also has some herself to boost her rapidly declining energy in order to face the task of cooking the meal of grilled salmon with sautéed vegetables and boiled new potatoes with white wine sauce for the family. Unfortunately, the sugar boost from the biscuits will only cause problems later on..

As soon as her husband Steve arrives, she feels she can 'let go' and 'drop some of the plates that she has been spinning in the air all day' without too many consequences. He plays with the kids whilst Susan tries to get dinner on the table. Susan would rather go straight to bed and let everyone eat and of course clean up after themselves. Her stress glands are pretty shattered at this point.

At the dinner table Susan eats her food at a hundred miles an hour and it does not even 'touch the sides'. Not chewing food properly can reduce the nutrient uptake from the meal and put stress on the

Not chewing food properly can reduce the nutrient uptake from the meal

digestive system. The kids play up (those biscuits were not such a great idea in the long run) but dad manages to keep them all entertained by his loud belching whilst at the same time inhaling his meal. The children do not finish their food (after all they did get a sugar fix beforehand) but Susan is too tired to encourage them to eat a little more.

Steve puts them to bed whilst Susan cleans up the dinner table and kitchen. At last, all is calm, Susan and Steve put their feet up with a glass of wine, whilst 'chatting' and watching the television. After a few sips of wine Susan has fallen asleep on the sofa and Steve tries to enjoy his programme on TV whilst his digestive system creates quite a 'ruckus' with some acid reflux and uncomfortable wind.

Susan has issues with energy which can partly be explained by her 'full on day' but also poor eating habits and Steve has digestive issues that are not helped with his marathon eating habits. We will see how Susan's energy improves dramatically but also the positive change in her children's behaviour.

Director dad...Richard

Director dad has high cholesterol and high blood pressure and feels he is doing very well on his new diet recommended by his doctor of avoiding butter, red meat, prawns, lobster and beer. Most of the foods that Richard has cut out actually contain the good fats apart from the beer.

Once he gets home, he greets the family, grabs a bag of reduced fat crisps and joins the kids in front of the TV. A few minutes later his partner shouts out to let him know his coffee is ready, black and no sugar...after all he is taking the dietary advice seriously.

What Richard is unaware of is that the reduced fat crisps contain the bad fats. Although he is no longer having sugar in his coffee, he does not realise that the coffee itself can increase his blood sugar levels as well as blood pressure and cholesterol. Richard had been given the option of taking some cholesterol lowering medication but decided to give the healthy eating approach a trial as he did not want the muscle twitching side effects that his golfing 'buddy' experienced along with lowered energy. We will see later how Richard did on the advice provided in this book.

the reduced fat crisps contain the bad fats

Girlfriend...Kate

Kate gets home from a busy full on day at work to her boyfriend playing computer games. Kate makes herself a herbal tea and grabs a beer for hopefully the husband-to-be. He takes a break for a few minutes to try and engage in her daily goings on as he wants to avoid another moody evening, she has just been having too many of those recently. These moody evenings started the same time as Kate started the diet.

As soon as his attention diminishes he turns back to the computer screen to get more of the adrenalin high that he is 'addicted' to. The computer games are constantly stimulating his adrenals which impact on his blood sugar levels without even eating.

Kate physically enjoys her herbal tea as she knows this is supposed to help her to fight off the stubborn fat around the tummy area, but mentally there is a roller coaster going on with her brain chemicals...she is craving chocolate cake but tries not to think about it by calling her mum for a chat before cooking the evening meal. The fat around the tummy area is also known as 'stress fat' and can

fat around the tummy area is also known as 'stress fat'

build up when blood sugar levels continuously spike up and down.

The 'boyfriend' does not even know what's for dinner let alone know how to cook and just enjoys his 'adrenaline high'. Kate's strong will and determination to lose this weight has got her cooking lower fat meals and she cooks an organic wheat free pasta dish with an organic tomato sauce containing at least three vegetables and a salad on the side, no wine, I did say she is strong willed and one day she will look 'perfect' in that 'wedding dress'. Kate's current diet is actually helping her to hold onto the weight as her blood sugar levels are also yo-yoing all day long. Her evening meal is a carbohydrate meal and lacks fat and protein which creates a blood sugar rush resulting in a lack of weight loss. We will see how Kate gets on later by adding protein and fat to each meal.

New mum...Gillie

Gillie is a new mum to a 9 week old baby boy. She has been on a course of antibiotics for mastitis and the baby (Jamie) was pretty easy going with no complaints until Jamie developed some kind of skin rash which Gillie noticed after the first vaccination. Her doctor reassures her that it is not linked to the vaccination and that newborns can have a few skin flare ups...all to do with the mother's hormones coming through the milk.

Gillie feels quite low at times, especially when she sees other mums from her ante-natal group looking like they have just walked out of a shoot from 'Hello' magazine. These ladies never seem to talk about anything of relevance to (her) life, she feels out of touch with them all, but does not speak up for fear of being 'unpopular' and losing her 'support' group. Gillie is exhausted most of the time, waking up at least 3-4 times in the night to feed. Her partner helps with one of the nightly feeds to give her some rest and he is worried about Gillie's recent personality changes since the birth. She seems to cry at the drop of a hat, has no energy to do anything. When he gets home from work she seems to be constantly 'whining' over petty issues.

During the day the overwhelming feeling of being 'in love' with her baby keeps her busy, she takes her baby to various classes during the week, from massage, swimming, baby yoga and music classes. These activities are suppose to 'benefit' the mental/emotional and physical development of her new love, as she keeps reading and hearing. However, her own health is of concern but her blood tests came back in the 'all clear'. This makes her feel even worse. At least a diagnosis would have confirmed that she is not going 'crazy'.

Gillie lost a considerable amount of hair during the final trimester of her pregnancy

Gillie lost a considerable amount of hair during the final trimester of her pregnancy and has lost even more since the birth but she keeps being told this is 'pretty normal' after pregnancy. Gillie is emotionally low and has been since the birth of Jamie. She may be suffering from postnatal depression and/or her nutritional habits may not be balanced. Is she balancing all main meals with the three food groups? Is she snacking in between, especially if the meals are more than 4 hours apart? And is she drinking enough water?

Single mum...Joanne

Joanne gets some financial help from the father of the children but only has just enough money to buy food for the week. She cooks all three meals a day religiously as it is cheaper but also healthier. The meals mainly consist of the staples: potato, pasta or bread. These foods load the blood with sugar pretty rapidly and therefore not as healthy as many people assume.

Her son has been diagnosed as having ADHD (Attention Deficit Hyperactivity Disorder) which is a behavioural developmental disorder but the thought of spending money on so-called 'healthy snacks' which are free from preservatives and colourings as suggested by a close friend costs as much as their lunch put together. ADHD usually presents in childhood and is characterised by persistent hyperactivity, inability to concentrate, forgetfulness, easily distracted and poor impulse control. Joanne's son's school headmaster has suggested that he may benefit from taking a medication called 'Ritalin', 'it can turn children around rather quickly' he tells her. But she has reservations, as she feels he is 'pretty normal at home'. Is he eating foods that are responsible for the ADHD symptoms? Is he unhappy at school?

has been diagnosed as having ADHD

Bulimic...Patricia

Patricia, a 32 year old social worker, has a pretty stressful job which is emotionally exhausting. This job in itself is impacting Patricia's blood sugar balance. By the time she gets home from work her blood sugar levels are so low that she is ravenous. Patricia eats two regular sized chocolate bars and within minutes of eating, throws up her food and takes two laxatives. This chocolate escalates her blood sugar and the laxatives not only 'rid' her body of food but also much needed minerals which are the spark plugs of our make up. Thirty minutes later she is feeling hungry (due to the plummeting blood sugar levels as the pancreas is now working with all its might to bring the sugar out of the blood stream) and cooks herself a grilled fish dish with steamed vegetables with no fat as she has already put on over seven kilos in the last year.

After dinner she is feeling lethargic and bloated and watches TV while flicking through a woman's magazine and an article about a 42-year old bulimic lawyer catches her eye. She is horrified to read that a woman can still be bulimic in her 40s.

About eight pm her friend calls to meet up, she declines saying she is not feeling well, but deep down she does not want to go out for fear of eating more calories. Not only is her bulimia playing havoc with her blood sugar levels but also intensifies her deeply unhappy emotional state. What sparked Patricia's bulimia? And how can she over-come this condition? We will see later that Patricia's blood sugar levels were balanced by implementing the Naked Truth lifestyle and the cause of her bulimia was successfully addressed.

she does not want to go out for fear of eating more calories

Anti-ageing grandmother...Mary

Mary ran a large PR firm before she retired and her husband still works as a City lawyer. She enjoys playing golf with the ladies at the club and likes to indulge in various pampering therapies as well as regular visits to the acupuncturist, nutritionist, herbalist and not to mention spending large sums of money on anti-ageing cosmetics. Mary has plenty of energy now that she has gone onto hormonal replacement therapy but more importantly (to her) it seems to be helping her to look younger. Her libido is still pretty non-existent which does not bother her much but her husband is getting worried and wonders about who exactly she plays golf with.

The hormone replacement therapy is only a short-term fix and when trying to achieve good health, short cuts do not pay off. We will see later that implementing the Naked Truth lifestyle and removing toxins from her life Mary helped herself considerably.

hormone replacement therapy is only a short-term fix

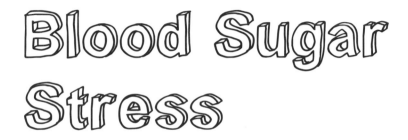

Blood Sugar Stress

In the next few pages I will introduce you to the adrenals also known as the stress glands and how important they are to the healthy running of our bodies.

These glands respond to stress that we experience daily. Stress can be physical or emotional and can cause ill health if the ability to adapt to it becomes weakened. This stress can be due to unhealthy nutritional lifestyle, surgery, unhappy marriage, unfulfilling job, etc.

Two prominent researchers, Hans Seyle and Claude Bernard were the founders of stress and the body's internal ability to adapt to change respectively.

Doctor Hans Seyle's Definition of Stress

Doctor Hans Seyle MD, PhD originated the concept of physiological stress. His definition of stress was 'the non-specific response of the body to any demand'. 'Any demand' being emotional demand or a physical demand. This includes, eating unhealthy foods, using toxic products such as household chemicals, unhappy marriage, the loss of a loved one etc. It could be anything that creates stress and it does not have to be something obvious like a tight deadline to finish a project. He was the first to propose that specific diseases, such as ulcers, immune fatigue, stroke, heart disease and nervous disorders could be related to the body's response to stress. It is vital that we do not forget these fundamental truths when building health.

Before this, it was believed that each disease had its own specific cause such as the example of heart disease being caused by high cholesterol, MRSA being caused by a multi-antibiotic resistant bug, diabetes being caused by high blood sugar. However, it is more complex than this. Dr. Seyle is saying that our body's response to ongoing stress can produce a range of diseases (as mentioned previously) which differ from person to person depending on the individual's susceptibility.

Claude Bernard's Theory

Louis Pasteur who is known for his 'germ theory' was quoted at the end of his life saying "Bernard was right, the microbe is nothing, the soil is everything". Bernard being Claude Bernard who was an eminent scientist. In essence, Claude was saying that it's not the bugs that are responsible for disease susceptibility but the health of the body (the soil)! If our body is healthy it can adapt and re-establish health, but if it is not healthy it is unable to adapt and thereby unable to re-establish health. For example, when the flu is 'going around' not everyone will get it as it depends on the overall health of the individual not just the presence of the flu causing microbe.

it's not the bugs that are responsible for disease susceptibility but the health of the body

This means that the phrase 'catching a cold' is incorrect. Why would you 'catch a cold' if your body is healthy? Surely your immune system would combat it effectively before it even had a chance to settle. However, if the body has been compromised such as by poor nutrition or surgery or emotional upset then the immune system is less likely to prevent the manifestation of a cold.

Understanding the basics of ongoing stress on the body and the vital importance of the health of the soil is pivotal in implementing the Naked Truth lifestyle.

The Adrenal Glands

The adrenal glands are our versatile stress glands. We have two of these glands. They respond to any stress be it emotional or physical. The adrenals DO NOT know the difference between real danger or perceived danger, they respond with the same 'vigour and vip' whether you have had a stimulant, viral infection, injury or stress at work. They are our basic 'survival' glands.

Picture our forefathers living out in the wild and hunting for food, when suddenly, a 'wild beast' appears. Their nervous system triggers the release of adrenaline by the adrenals. Adrenaline is our primary stress hormone. The adrenaline promptly and efficiently increases blood sugar levels which provides instant fuel allowing these hunters to run for their lives. Without this adrenaline surge these men would be more or less savaged by the beast. On running for their lives they burn off the blood sugar and come to a safe place. The adrenals no longer sense the danger and the blood sugar levels drop back to normal.

It is very important to note that the adrenals do their job by primarily providing instant fuel to escape (and by raising the heart rate, perspiration etc - all equally important functions) and the hunters then burn off the sugar fuel as they run for their life to safety. So the sugar doesn't remain in the bloodstream to cause damage to the internal workings of the body.

The Twenty First Century Adrenal Status

In today's society it is a different picture for the adrenals all together. Remember I mentioned that the adrenals do not know the difference between real danger OR perceived danger? Unlike our ancestors who faced life or death situations on a regular basis the dangers in our lives today are more subtle but have the same long-term impact on our adrenal glands. Let me tell you about what some of these dangers are:

1. junk food: fast food; croissants, bagels, cakes, biscuits, coffee, alcohol, drugs
2. emotional dangers: stress of work, grief, long-term unhappiness, loneliness, shock, depression, anger, lack of fulfilment
3. physical trauma such as an accident or surgery
4. biological toxins: viral infections, bacterial infections, fungal infections etc
5. chemical toxins: pesticides, drugs, vaccinations, household chemicals, medical drugs

Real or perceived dangers create the same adrenal response as does the 'wild beast in the hunter gatherer'. Let's analyse what's going on internally when we rush off to work without breakfast and grab a coffee and a croissant on the way.

The coffee stimulates the adrenals to release adrenaline which creates the blood sugar surge...to add insult to injury the white flour and sugar in the croissant create a blood sugar increase as well. This major sugar 'overload' gets the pancreas (a gland that ensures sugar does not stay at high levels in the blood in order to protect the body from becoming ill) throwing out insulin as if life or death depended on it (which it does when we consider, insulin resistance, heart disease, diabetes, glaucoma, kidney malfunction etc). The end result is to bring the blood sugar down (in other words out of the blood into the cells). At this time, we

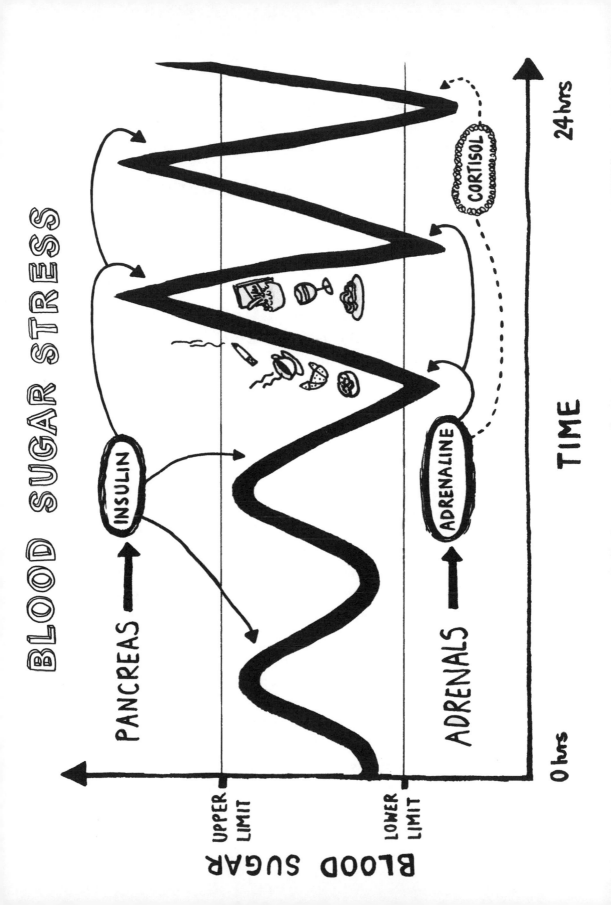

do not think, 'oh wait, I have just had a coffee which has released sugar in my system let me run around the block to burn off the sugar surge'. So the body has a natural mechanism to stop too much blood sugar hanging around and causing damage. However, our modern lifestyles are playing havoc with this vital mechanism.

When this blood sugar 'yo-yoing' has been going on for a while, the body can start to become less sensitive to its own insulin, thereby allowing sugar to remain in the blood. This can lead to conditions varying from insulin resistance, weight gain, diabetes, high blood pressure, anxiety, mood swings, cancer, not to mention speeding up the ageing process! ..so the grandmother, Mary, can do all the therapies she likes as well as intoxicate her body with synthetic hormones, but her blood sugar 'yo-yoing' can create what we call 'free radicals' (also known as oxidants) which cause damage to cells and speed up ageing.

the body has a natural mechanism to stop too much blood sugar hanging around and causing damage. However, our modern lifestyles are playing havoc with this vital mechanism

Even skipping meals can bring blood sugar levels down too low. Lowered blood sugar sends a message to the adrenals that your life is in danger which triggers the adrenaline surge and so the cycle begins....what a roller-coaster ride!

When this adrenal stress is on-going, such as poor nutrition not balanced with all food groups, a stressful job, continuous ill health, unhappy home life, etc the main job of adrenaline from the adrenals is taken over by a hormone called 'cortisol'.

Cortisol is the long-term version of adrenaline (adrenaline should do its job within a few minutes, by that time the stress should have been removed!) But in today's world stress is continuous and takes its toll on the body. It is like the cortisol has to take the 'flak' because adrenaline is short acting. Now cortisol in balance is 'perfect' for great health, but if levels are too high or too low then we can experience all sorts of unhealthy symptoms. The following are just a few of them:

- Heart disease
- High blood pressure
- Weight gain around stomach area
- Digestive disturbances: irritable bowel, flatulence, bloating, excessive belching
- Candida – fungal infection
- High levels of toxic fats
- Skin problems: acne, rapid ageing
- Menstrual problems example unexplained infertility
- Diabetes
- Food intolerances
- Hay fever
- Weight gain
- Sluggish thyroid
- Behavioural imbalances such as poor memory, depression
- General swelling –'puffiness' (usually called oedema)
- Arthritis
- Chronic fatigue

Having all three food groups in each meal is pretty important because by doing this you are preventing such blood sugar surges. The intricate balance of important minerals such as sodium, magnesium and potassium (to name a few) becomes imbalanced during prolonged adrenal activity. These minerals are absolutely vital in achieving optimum health – they are the spark plugs of our biochemistry.

As I have mentioned minerals, I would like to add at this point that one should avoid standard table salt and use the non refined salt like the Himalayan salt or the Celtic sea salt. Standard table salt is basically sodium chloride whereas non refined salt contains a whole range of minerals that are found in the body. Table salt was originally made for manufacturing products such as PVC not for human consumption! Stick with the real salt and use it daily. This unrefined salt does not negatively impact blood pressure. This wholesome salt is important in helping regulate blood pressure as well as regulating other physiological processes.

So what are the benefits of maintaining healthy blood sugar levels? The following are what I call the tip of the iceberg improvements – what happens below the iceberg is of utmost importance too.

- **Weight loss**
- **Sharper mind and better memory**
- **Increased energy**
- **Healthier immune system**
- **Balanced blood pressure**
- **Better digestion**
- **Reduced toxic fats**
- **Improved liver function**
- **Calmer mind**
- **Hormonal balance**
- **Anti-ageing**
- **Improved libido**
- **Reduced 'allergies'**

Twenty First Century Babies

This on-going situation is getting so extreme that even babies are beginning to be born with these symptoms. They are being born with adrenals that are already partially 'tired'. The newborn symptoms may include:

- colic
- acid reflux
- eczema
- diabetes
- difficulty sleeping
- not feeding well
- blocked/loose bowels

There are more 'medicalised' births, as the mother's adrenals are in 'over-drive'. When adrenaline or cortisol is in the blood stream, the body will either not give birth or it will slow down the labour process. Why? Because the body will not give birth if the message it is receiving is 'run, I am in danger, the beast is after my life'.

The mother's feelings about the birth or during the birth are of utmost importance. Is she stressed, fearful or anxious of giving birth? When this is the case the adrenals are picking up 'danger' and the body goes into 'survival' mode which makes it impossible for the mother to give birth naturally. In such cases drugs are introduced to so-call 'progress' the labour or surgery becomes necessary. Whichever course of action is taken the baby is 'frightened' to come out as it has picked up the 'danger' signals from mum's adrenals.

There are more 'medicalised' births, as the mother's adrenals are in 'over-drive'

The new born can come out in a state of 'shock' and can live with this 'shock' for the rest of his/her life. It is important that the mother's state of health before, during and after birth is considered. The 'shock' in the baby and also in the mother can be remedied by various approaches such as counselling for the mother, homeopathy and/or cranial osteopathy for mother and baby. This may all sound a bit dramatic but this is the way the body works. We are wired for survival be it with or without ill health.

The baby can present with anxiety, irritability, develop bad sleeping habits, colic, acid reflux, failure to thrive (not absorb their nutrients) constipation, kidney issues or inability to breast feed (due to the internal subconscious 'fight or flight' message). Essentially they are in hyper vigilant mode. Living lifestyles of adrenaline and cortisol highs and lows not only impacts our own health but the health of our children.

The baby can present with anxiety, irritability, develop bad sleeping habits, colic, acid reflux, failure to thrive

The Gut

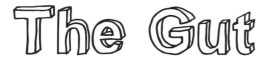

It is very important that our body turns our food into the basic nutrients that it can use therefore it is important that our digestive system is healthy.

Hippocrates, the father of medicine from ancient Greece is known for saying 'all diseases begin in the gut' but he was around in 460-370 BC at which time life was different to our fast paced culture. The adrenals play a critical role in the health of the gut. If the adrenals are constantly 'on the go' they reduce the ability of the gut to turn our food into basic nutrients.

The digestive system is one of the most utilised systems in our body. After all we eat at least three times a day whether it is healthy or not. There are various important processes that need to be fully functional within the digestive system otherwise all the healthy eating, healthy supplement 'taking', healthy exercising etc will not address our health concerns. The role of the digestive system is to process the food into its basic goodness. So how do we optimise our digestion?

The first important process is CHEWING food and not rushing it. When food is chewed the amazing enzymes in the saliva start the process of breaking down the food. As the mouth chews, the stomach is preparing to receive the food for further digestion by releasing acid.

The second process is digestion of the food in the stomach. The acidity within the stomach is of great importance. Not only does it kill the bugs on or within the food, the acid further digests the food to enable it to pass downstream to the gut. Without enough stomach acidity we are unable to extract the nutrients (specifically the minerals) from our food, so we can become nutrient depleted, resulting in any manner of symptoms from hair loss through to diabetes.

Once the stomach has done its job, the food is passed down the gut where the third process begins. The third process involves pancreatic enzymes, the alkaline juice and bile from the liver. This process further digests the food into its smallest units before it is finally absorbed.

The fourth process is the absorption of the digested food which moves into the blood stream and is further processed according to the body's needs at that time.

Adrenal-Gut Relationship

When we are stressed the important acidity in the stomach reduces. WHY? Because our body is 'running' from the life threatening danger so conserving all energy to 'fight or flee'. As the body needs all it's energy to fight or flee then this is diverted away from the digestive system which then slows down. The cortisol (the long term stress hormone) in the blood stream triggers various digestive changes, these include:

- **reduction in stomach acid**
- **reduction in the digestive enzymes**
- **re-routing of the blood from the digestive system to the main muscles (to fight or flee)**
- **general slowing down of the heal and repair processes in the body which the digestive system especially requires daily**

As soon as our stomach acidity reduces we are no longer able to absorb all the goodness from what we eat, especially the minerals. Furthermore, a reduction in stomach acid hinders the pancreas from releasing much of the alkaline juice or the enzymes. There has to be a certain amount of acidity coming from the stomach to 'trigger' the pancreas to release its alkaline juice with the various digestive enzymes. In other words with a poor second stage of the digestive process the third stage will be impaired. All in all this prevents our body from obtaining the 'goodness' from our food. Reduced stomach acidity also hinders the immune system.

imagine, living under ongoing stress, not only do we stock up on stimulants to keep us going which are nutrient robbers in themselves, but our digestive system starts shutting down too

So imagine, living under ongoing stress (very much a twenty first century lifestyle), not only do we stock up on stimulants to keep us going which are nutrient robbers in themselves, but our digestive system starts shutting down too resulting in further nutrient depletion.

Leaky Gut

In some cases the cortisol can inflame the digestive system which results in what is known as a 'leaky' gut. A 'leaky' gut is basically the equivalent of a hose pipe punctured with small holes. Such a hose pipe would leak out water where it should not and the same applies to the 'leaky' gut. Before the food is completely digested it leaks out into the blood stream and this can result in any of the following symptoms:

- bloating
- food intolerances/allergies
- hay fever
- diarrhoea

- skin problems: eczema, acne
- hair loss
- loss of muscle
- lethargy
- brain 'fog'
- food cravings
- a lowered immune system; re-occurring cold/flu, chest infections etc

One of the most common symptoms of a leaky gut is the systemic fungal infection, Candida. Candida is a symptom of an underlying imbalance. By solely addressing the diet to starve the Candida (which is yeast, sugar, wheat, dairy and vinegar free) is again like inflating a punctured car tyre. The so-called Candida diet is not an easy one to follow as when you have a small treat, the symptoms usually flare up! Candida is a fungus that we all have internally, but it is only when the body's soil has been disrupted that it will grow out of balance and create a plethora of symptoms. So many of our illnesses are a reflection of an underlying imbalance. The damaging effects of a 'leaky' gut are endless, all due to the 'fight or flight' response in this case.

It is worth considering that a 'leaky' gut can also occur through antibiotic use, consuming foods that one is intolerant to, steroid medications, to name just a few.

It can be beneficial to take some natural digestive aids (see Getting Going chapter later) in order to support the gut when suffering from adrenal stress otherwise you can just end up spending a considerable amount of money just 'chasing' symptoms by not addressing the cause.

It is generally believed that Candida thrives in an acidic environment but again there are no short cuts as some people may be tempted to alkalinise their body (in other words reduce

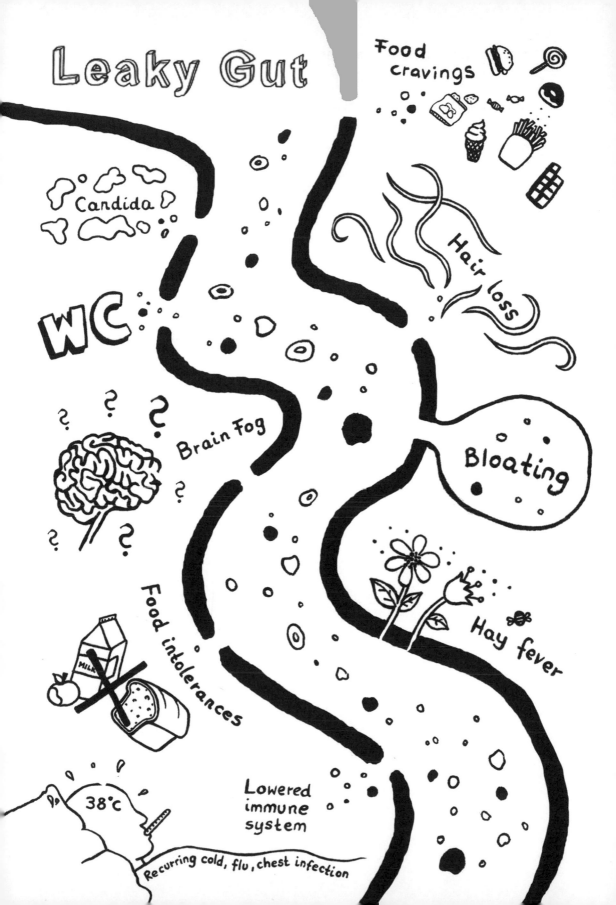

the acidity) for example by drinking alkalinising water. We need our stomach's strong acidity to digest food but also to absorb minerals. The stomach is unable to do this if its acidity is being 'neutralised' by such alkalinising methods. In other words it is important to address the cause of a symptom and not just dampen the symptom.

a 'leaky' gut can also occur through antibiotic use, consuming foods that one is intolerant to, steroid medications, to name just a few

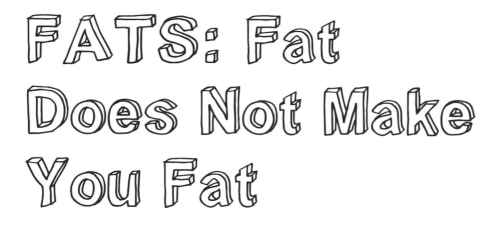

FATS: Fat Does Not Make You Fat

Cholesterol Craze

People are advised to cut down on eggs, red meat, butter, cream and various sea foods and switch to low fat foods when they have been diagnosed with high cholesterol.

I believe before taking on this advice, one should ask a few common sense questions:

- What is the role of cholesterol?
- Why is the cholesterol high?
- Would cutting out foods that are natural be of benefit in the long term?
- Is my medication addressing the 'cause' of my ill health?
- What can I do to improve my health, so balancing my cholesterol?

So what is the answer to cholesterol?

In order to answer this question, we need to familiarise our selves with the 'diet-heart hypothesis' in chapter two which suggested that if we eat cholesterol and/or saturated fats our arteries will become clogged by so-called plaques with resulting high blood pressure, heart attacks or stroke.

Cholesterol was blamed for this as it was found in the artery-clogging plaque. So the logic went that if the 'plaquing' (if there is such a word) is causing all the harm and cholesterol is found in this 'plaque', well the cause must be the cholesterol. BINGO! And the cholesterol lowering drugs were produced in their masses in all their 'glory'.

Well, I just want to stop here and give a more truthful version of the plaquing process. When the lining of the artery wall is damaged/injured this triggers a whole host of events known as inflammation – primarily the immune cells (known as white blood cells) arrive at the site of injury and start to clear up the mess. The injury also 'calls out' other healing agents to help in repairing the damage and

A scar forms which is the manifestation of a healed wound and the job is done

cholesterol is one of the agents. A scar forms which is the manifestation of a healed wound and the job is done.

However, in today's society we have ongoing damage to the artery walls, so in effect the body is constantly trying to heal and repair this damage. So instead of a nice neat scar being formed an 'atherosclerotic plaque' is formed which in simple terms is an 'unhealed scar'. This 'unhealed scar' can rupture anytime which creates a blood clot that narrows the artery. Also there is the risk that this blood clot will dislodge and travel down blood vessels such as the blood vessel that supplies the brain and which then leads to a stroke.

You may ask why the scar does not heal? Well that is because the original damage that triggers inflammation has not been addressed appropriately, so the inflammation continues without any boundaries.

So the important question here is what damages the artery walls in the first place to trigger inflammation? The damage can be created by a number of factors and these include:

- **Cortisol a stress hormone which can be inflammatory (so that may be the reason why most heart attacks occur on a Monday morning!)**
- **Smoking**
- **Hydrogenated fats also known as trans fats**
- **Caffeine**
- **Sugar**
- **Infections**

Please note the list does not contain saturated fats or cholesterol for that matter.

One thing all the above causal factors have in common is inflammation (the body's response to injury). Inflammation when controlled (for example through a healthy lifestyle) is vital for healing but if the inflammation is ongoing and does not resolve (for example in the constant presence of any of the above factors), this not only creates further damage to the arterial wall but also can create all sorts of other mischief.

Cholesterol is made by the liver which is the largest organ inside our body. The liver also plays a major role in metabolism, digestion, detoxification and the elimination of toxins from the body.

The liver makes more cholesterol when there is damage to the body. Imagine the liver as a cholesterol thermostat. Most of our cholesterol comes from within and not without as most of us are led to believe. So when one has an X amount of cholesterol coming through their diet, a healthy functioning liver will register that and accommodate for that. For example if the diet that day was rich in so-called cholesterol foods such as red meat or full fat cheese, then the liver will register that and make less cholesterol that day. If however more cholesterol is required that day, may be due to less being consumed or stress such as damage to the body (which can be internal or external damage) then the liver will make more cholesterol on that day. So it is also vital to have a healthy functioning liver to regulate our cholesterol levels.

Cholesterol is Vital

So what exactly is the role of cholesterol in our bodies? Are you ready for this? You may just want sit down. Cholesterol is found in every cell – without it the cell would not function, and it is vital in the repair process.

Other important roles of cholesterol in the body include:

- **boosting mental performance**
- **keeping the cells intact**
- **maintaining your energy, vitality, libido and fertility**
- **helps digestion**
- **builds strong bones**
- **builds muscle**
- **regulates your blood sugar**
- **repairs damage in the body**
- **protects against infectious diseases**
- **helps with clearing the body from toxins**

Another very important point is that your stress hormone cortisol is made from cholesterol, so that 'stressful' events such as putting a cuff around the arm prior to taking a blood sample or fear of a needle can result in raised cholesterol values!

If we reduce cholesterol using drugs then how is the body going to be able to make cortisol in order to cope with stress and how will the body heal and repair cells?

Perhaps by throwing a 'wobbly' and creating another symptom such as a heart attack? In other words blocking the body's natural healing mechanisms is not the answer.

stress hormone cortisol is made from cholesterol

Your body is a complex being and trying to address a symptom such as high cholesterol rather than the ongoing underlying cause is harmful in the long term.

Scientific research is showing that so-called cholesterol lowering medications do not reduce the incidence of heart disease by lowering cholesterol but by reducing inflammation! As mentioned earlier, inflammation is triggered by a number of factors including adrenaline, cortisol, caffeine, sugar, rancid fats etc. So why not remove these inflammation creating triggers and thereby avoiding un-necessary medication?

So Richard the director dad wisely chose to change his diet, irrespective of his high cholesterol. His diet however, is not 'health promoting' therefore it will continue to have a negative impact on his 'health' because he is in the 'adrenal over-drive' zone. His coffee when he gets home starts that crazy adrenaline triggered blood sugar spiral. The adrenals also depend on a good liver to help them along their role in life. So when the adrenals are constantly calling on the liver for help (as the adrenals do whenever they are triggered), the liver gets over burdened and is unable to regulate cholesterol levels efficiently. So the first bit of advice for Richard was to cut out all coffee and low fat 'foods' (like his crisps). Caffeine is a well known 'toxin' which has to be cleared/detoxed by the liver, so cutting down on coffee is very beneficial as not only does it reduce the workload on the liver but also the adrenals.

The liver can get pretty unhappy when exposed to toxins such as hydrogenated fats, medications, refined carbohydrates and stimulants such as alcohol and caffeine. In basic terms the liver gets over-burdened and needs help in reducing this burden. Taking out natural foods (like red meat, butter, cream) is not the answer. So that leads onto another question...if we are stressed and the body requires more cortisol to 'deal' with the stress, then the liver would have to provide more cholesterol in order to make more of the stress hormone cortisol...right? Then why reduce cholesterol if it is part of our survival mechanism not harming mechanism?

The body through the liver is 'crying out for help' and what we seem to do with cholesterol lowering drugs or the low fat diet is 'drown' out the cry for a while, for the cry to only get louder later.

The cholesterol story is not this simple but the basic importance and mis-information on cholesterol has hopefully been high lighted.

So let's address the root cause by helping out the liver as well as cleaning up the nutritional intake.

Richard the director dad

When Richard came to see me, I saw that he was a very hard working, driven and determined man. His mortgage and more was very much dependent on his financial income. He was a pretty straight forward 'no messing, lets get on with it' kind of individual. His main goal was to reduce his cholesterol until I explained the important healing role of cholesterol and that it is not the villain it has been made out to be.

When I first recommended the Naked Truth lifestyle he was alarmed and a little uncomfortable about being advised that eating red meat and butter was absolutely fine. He had some very good questions, as to the why's and how's of the Naked Truth lifestyle. He was astounded by

one of his colleagues was always getting migraines, until he gave up his 'diet coke' habit.

the information I gave him on artificial sweeteners although he did comment that one of his colleagues was always getting migraines, until he gave up his 'diet coke' habit.

I advised that he:

1. clean up his diet and implement the Naked Truth lifestyle with healthy snacks in between his meals
2. take some nutritional/herbal supplements (see Getting Going chapter later) to support his adrenals and liver
3. remove all hydrogenated fats
4. reduce stress, so that the adrenals can also back off from draining the liver's energy

Richard followed everything to the 'letter' and his cholesterol went back within the 'normal' range, lost weight and he also commented on having more mental clarity and physical energy.

At his follow up session I noticed his skin was clearer and he actually 'sat back in the chair' rather than sit on the edge of it, as if ready to 'fight or flight' as he did in the first session. He had also decided on seeing a 'life coach' to help him to manage his stress better.

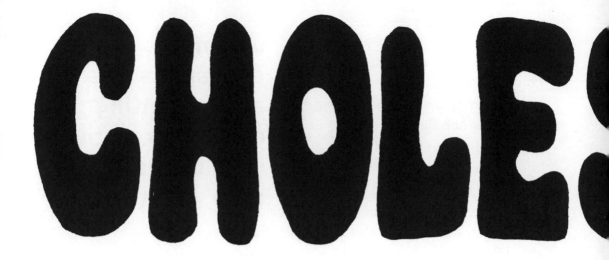

CHOLES

... IT'S ESSENTIAL

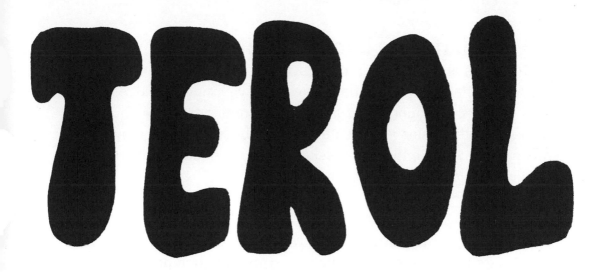

VITALITY

BONES

HEALING

IMMUNITY

Fats that have been exploited

Toxic fats or bad fats are totally synthetic. You will not find them in nature however hard you try. As you may have guessed, if they are not found in nature then consuming them will not help in addressing your health issues. These toxic fats play an important role in the progression of various health problems including obesity and heart disease.

These fats are generally found in 'low fat' foods, they are also known as hydrogenated fats or trans fats. Hydrogenated fats are fats that have been through the hydrogenation process. The purpose of this is to solidify oils so that they can be made to resemble real foods such as butter. In addition they are cheaper to produce, have a 'desirable texture' and have a longer shelf life. We all know fresh food goes off quickly. So why not buy butter instead of margarine?

Damaging impact of synthetic fats

These synthetic fats are NOT recognised by the body and so they conveniently manage to 'slip' into the cell membrane. Without becoming a 'jargon' junkie, the cell membrane has many important functions but I am just focusing on its role as a semi-permeable skin layer around the cell. This layer keeps the cellular environment 'healthy' (the junk out and the goodness in). The cell membrane is vital for cell to cell communication. Cells 'speak' to each other like we speak with one another. Without communication we fail, so does the cell and hence the body.

Imagine a regular conversation with your best friend...you're excited and share your news and they share theirs using their hands and facial expressions or any other gestures that they like. Now try having a conversation with your best friend with your hands 'tied back' and slightly intoxicated with alcohol. Your conversation will be somewhat fuzzy. The same is true when these hydrogenated fats are present in your cells – 'their hands are tied back' which impedes communication between the cells and hence between various organs (such as adrenals, liver, pancreas etc) and systems in the body (such as respiratory, reproductive, detox symptoms etc). All organs are made from cells and all systems are made from organs. So just to

try having a conversation with your best friend with your hands 'tied back' and slightly intoxicated with alcohol

repeat all organs are made from cells and all systems are made from organs. So we need to nourish the cell membrane with 'goodness'.

Richard would do much better by avoiding his 'low fat' foods as well as coffee and eating as much natural food as possible. Coming home to a cup of herbal tea with a handful of nuts and seeds, whilst entertaining the kids would do him the 'world of good'.

Kate's toxic fats

Kate is someone who has battled with her weight since her teens. She has had a dominating father and a rather 'submissive' mother. She was told by her mother from a young age, 'that men only go for slim girls nowadays' and ended up in a 'career' because of her father's influence, rather than her own desires. She had been through every diet that I had come across and more! Initially she did incredibly well on these diets and managed to even get back to her size 10, but over the years her weight plateaued at size 14, even the starvation 'diet' did not work anymore.

Kate's adrenals and pancreas were trying their best to manage the blood sugar circus act created by the yo-yo dieting as well as her current low protein and low fat diet. Her body thought she was in danger (due to her high and low blood sugar levels created by the restrictive eating) and starts storing energy from the carbohydrate meals in the form of fat. As she avoids eating snacks her blood sugar drops too low therefore on a subconscious level her body does not know when she will find the next meal and so escape this 'perceived' danger (we're going back to the hunter gatherer days of our ancestors). For this reason her metabolism goes into storage mode. The body thinks it is better to store the calories than burn them off in times of danger!

To further add insult to injury, Kate's imbalanced cortisol levels were preventing the thyroid from working at its best which slows down her metabolism even further (cortisol slows down the thyroid in order to reserve energy to 'run' and not for good old metabolism that's regulated by the thyroid).

One of Kate's biggest battles was trying to fight off the last few pounds of fat around the abdominal area. This fat is called 'stress fat'. If you are struggling to lose that layer around the abdomen then ask yourself whether your adrenals are over working? If your meals are not balanced with all three food groups and you are consuming stimulants then the answer is 'yes'. Therefore the adrenals would do well with some nourishment and support (see Get Going chapter later).

After Kate saw me, she followed the Naked Truth lifestyle and took some supplements to support her adrenals. Without these she would not be able to fight off the 'cushion of fat' around her abdomen. Her cortisol levels came down within three weeks and she had lost enough weight to go down to a size 12. Kate lost not only her weight but her mood swings also improved by the third session which was three months following her first session.

By understanding that our adrenals also feed off our mental/
emotional state, Kate sought help from a psychotherapist to
help deal with her low self-esteem. She soon realised that
losing weight was not going to change her boyfriend into a
caring and communicative person and so she moved on.

Something that I notice quite often in practice amongst
individuals who yo-yo diet on low fat diets, is the slowing down
of their overall metabolism. This is indicated by the fact that
they can no longer lose weight on calorie restricted diets. This
generally creates a vicious cycle of weight loss and then weight
gain. Unfortunately the weight gain following weight loss is
usually more than the original loss.

**slowing down of
the metabolism in
individuals who
yo-yo diet**

Artificial Sweeteners: Not So Sweet

Artificial sweeteners containing the toxic aspartame also known as E951 seem to be incredibly popular amongst the 'weight conscious'.

However, I am not sure how many people using this so-called alternative to calorie laden sugar know that the FDA (Food and Drug Administration) in the USA has received more complaints about the side effects of aspartame than any other food ingredient. Aspartame is marketed under a number of trademark names, including Canderel, Equal and NutraSweet. It is commonly used in diet drinks, some ready made meals (more so the low-fat ones) sugar-free chewing gums, breath mints and low-fat yoghurts. It is also present in some medications. It is pretty 'shocking' how much 'rubbish' goes into some of our 'foods' so always read the label.

Aspartame is popular amongst diabetics and 'dieters' as they are led to believe it is safe, but it still creates an insulin surge just like sweet old sugar and has actually been linked to diabetes. I have seen patients get well just by giving up this toxic substitute. Aspartame is known to inhibit various brain chemicals, one of them being the well-known happy molecule called 'serotonin'. One study which looked into the effects of aspartame in depressed individuals actually had to be stopped because some of the individuals started to experience memory loss, others became more depressed or irritable and some started having nightmares. Other synthetic sweeteners that hinder good health include saccharin and sucralose.

As I do not want to advocate a strict regime of no 'fun' or 'treat' foods, you can use xylitol as a sugar substitute. Xylitol comes from a natural source and depending upon the brand it can vary as to where it is from. It is basically found in fruits such as plums and pineapples and does not have the same blood sugar surging effect as regular table sugar or the potential to increase fatty liver as fructose does and not to forget to mention it does not have the aspartame toxicity.

I do not want to advocate a strict regime of no 'fun' or 'treat' foods

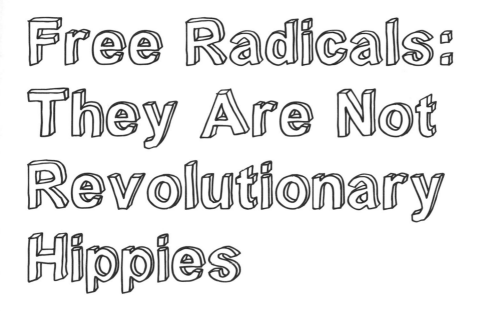

Free Radicals: They Are Not Revolutionary Hippies

Now this is not some kind of rock band and I am not side tracking at all. Without getting too 'jargon' based on you, a free radical is a chemical species in the body with an unpaired electron in the outer orbit.

All this means, is that a free radical is lonely and it basically will do anything to find itself a partner (known as an electron). It will do this by stealing an electron from another source which then creates more free radicals (from the source it 'stole' from, theft I call it!). This just escalates out of proportion especially if the free radical steals from our genetic material or the membranes protecting the cells.

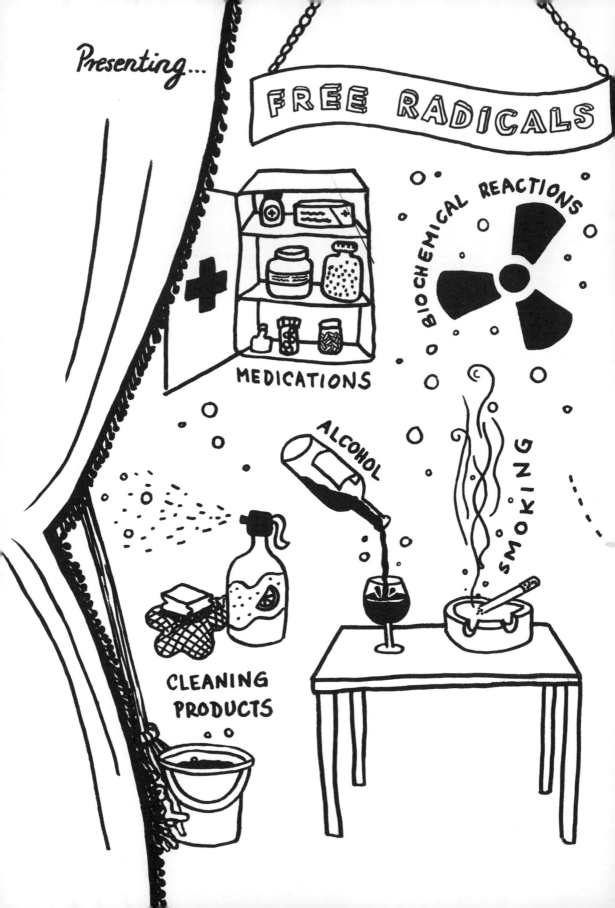

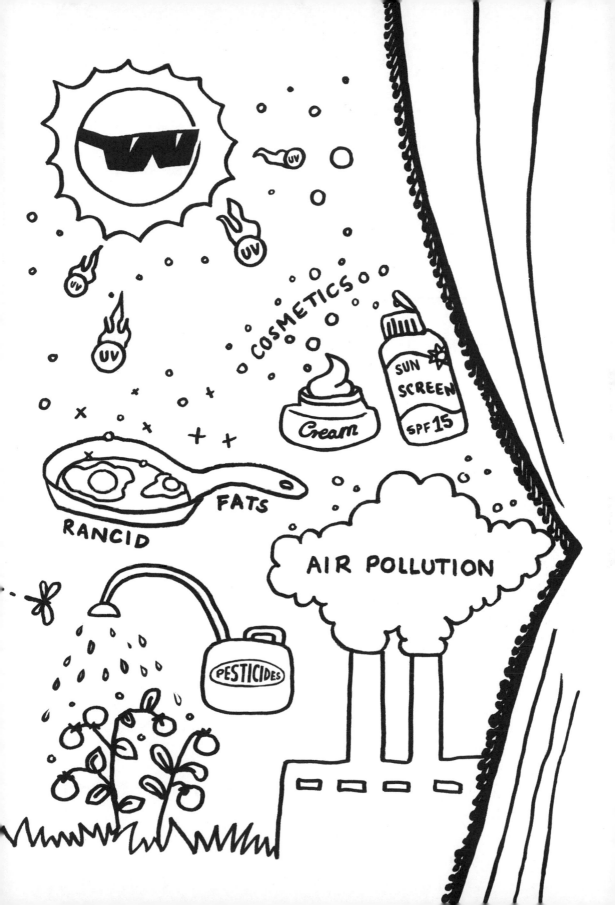

When the adrenals are stressed – especially on an ongoing basis – cortisol can create these harmful free radicals. Taking good care of the adrenals is a huge start in preventing mass free radical production. Free radicals are also produced during:

- cleaning up everyday toxins
- injury
- strenuous activity
- various biochemical reactions
- immune system activation

Free radicals can also be produced from outside sources such as:

- air pollution
- cigarette smoking
- excessive alcohol intake
- UV radiation
- pesticides
- medications
- hydrogenated fats
- certain cosmetic products

Cooking with polyunsaturated oils, which are oils that have several carbon-carbon double bonds such as sunflower oil, vegetable oil or canola oil produces rancid fats – in other words free radicals. We should be cooking with either saturated fats such as butter, coconut oil, palm oil or olive oil if cooking at lower temperatures. Saturated fats are stable when heated and monounsaturated fats like olive oil that have one carbon-carbon double bond are not as stable as saturated fats at higher temperatures.

Finally 'excited' adrenal glands themselves can also be a source of these 'scavenging' agents.

Free radicals can lead to numerous health issues from heart disease through to Alzheimer's with the help of other factors like poor diet, stress, depression etc. We can also take a good anti-oxidant to help quench the free radicals as well as removing them as much as possible from our lifestyles.

The Acid-Alkaline Theory

The mention of free radicals brings me onto the acid alkaline theory because ongoing accumulation of free radicals is known to create an acidic environment in the body. Allow me to expand on this theory.

In general there has been quite a buzz around boosting health and eliminating 'disease' by alkalinising the body. Basically this means shifting the pH of the body to a slightly higher level because it is believed that an alkaline system can not 'harbour' illnesses. Although this has some truth, the 'pitfall' with this is that our bodies actually swing from an acid pH to an alkaline pH on a daily basis, it is known as our circadian rhythm.

We are alkaline when we are in 'rest and digest mode' which is basically when we are in 'healing' mode and we are acidic when we are in 'fight or flight mode'. The other time when our system can become 'stuck' in acidity is when our detox organs are over-burdened. These detox organs include, the skin, lungs, liver, kidneys, bladder and bowels.

What puts stress on our detox organs? Well all the factors mentioned in the blood sugar stress chapter impact our detox organs which are junk foods, emotional stress, physical trauma, biological and chemical toxins. Not to mention that adrenaline, cortisol and sugar are acidifying.

When the above factors are continuous or ongoing (in other words not being addressed) then the pH of our system will drop in other words become more acidic. If our detox organs are working optimally and we implemented the Naked Health lifestyle we would not have to deal with being stuck in 'acidity'.

So the answer is not to just 'dampen' the acidity by using alkalinising powders and such like (a short-term fix) but to address the health of the detox organs and follow the Naked Truth lifestyle.

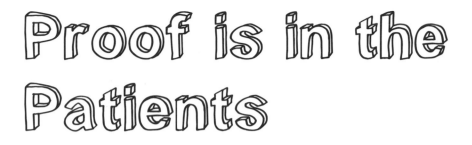

Proof is in the Patients

Susan...the exhausted mother

When Susan came to see me she was exhausted and pretty emotional. She felt that her life was on a conveyer belt and she just could not stop it.

She was no longer sleeping through the night and when she did manage to fall into a deep sleep it was time to wake up. Her legs felt like 'lead' in the mornings and she literally was being 'dragged' out of bed by her children. If she had the choice she would sleep all day and more.

Her diet was as follows:

Breakfast: marmalade on wholegrain toast or some kind of cereal (many cereals contain sugar) with semi-skimmed milk and a cup of Earl Grey tea

Lunch: sandwich, usually ham with some lettuce, tomato and cheese (whatever was in the fridge) with fruit juice

Dinner: four out of the seven evenings she cooked from scratch, the other evenings she had quick dinners like a pizza.

Nutritional changes

Yes, it is a cliché but breakfast is the most important meal of the day. By eating a 'junky' breakfast, you are heading for the adrenal roller coaster ride. When Susan introduced the Naked Truth lifestyle within a few days she noticed improvement in her energy levels and over the next few months she was sleeping better and even had the energy in the evenings to join her local 'book club'.

By eating a 'junky' breakfast, you are heading for the adrenal roller coaster ride

One of the most important changes that Susan made was to add two snacks into her daily lifestyle as well as removing the stimulants such as Earl Grey tea. Her snacks ALWAYS included a carbohydrate with EITHER a protein or fat. She went from having her tea and biscuits to having any of the following:

- **spelt crackers with humus**
- **almond butter with banana**
- **cheese with grapes**
- **apple with a handful of almonds and pumpkin seeds**
- **PLAIN yoghurt with a few tablespoons of her 1.5 yr olds pureed pear**
- **Protein shake**

No more 'junk' meant no more ....

Processed fruit juice
Marmalade
Biscuits
Tea
Pizza
Oven fries
Nuggets

Her children followed the same nutritional lifestyle and both Susan and her husband noticed changes in their children's behaviour especially in the evenings. There was a lot less fighting and 'destroying' the house was something of the past.

Susan's marriage also improved. She no longer fell asleep in front of the TV after sedating herself with wine. She commented that her libido was back to more or less to what it was before she had the children.

Susan also needed to 'get out of the house' and do something for herself. Since she became a mother she felt that she had lost her identity. She no longer felt that she was 'interesting' as all she could talk about was her 'exhausting life' and her children – she had no time to do anything else.

It would have been pretty ridiculous to ask a full-time mother, whose husband works long hours to find some time to pursue a 'hobby' in order to find time for herself. She would have laughed if I had suggested it at the first session. But as her energy levels increased and she no longer experienced the 'lows and highs' she decided to find interests for herself. She has now started a course to embark on a new career.

Gillie...the new mum

Gillie ran her own business as an interior designer with her business partner before she fell pregnant. She decided to take time out of the business in the middle of her second trimester as she felt that she was getting a bit 'run down' and wanted to prepare for a healthy natural birth. During her pregnancy Gillie had decided to become a vegetarian as she could not 'face' the smell of meat. She had always done well on meat protein but just could not face it at this time. Gillie felt great in the first trimester and third trimester but the second trimester was pretty exhausting. She had a tiring birth but it all went well. In herself she felt that after the birth 'something happened'. She became slightly anxious, was losing more hair and felt 'depressed'. She could not tolerate the 'mothers' in her ante natal group anymore and would 'flip' with her husband over 'petty' things like leaving the toothpaste tube open. Gillie knew this was not 'normal' for her.

mood swings disappeared as soon as she included protein

Having taken antibiotics (for the mastitis), she took a good probiotic to address the bacteria in the gut. She was on various supplements for the thyroid and she always ensured that she ate three square meals a day, although she did not include protein at every meal – because it was just too much work.

On taking her case history, it came to light she was very low on protein as well as stomach acid. The thyroid (as well as the adrenals) just 'loves' protein, so she adopted the Naked Truth lifestyle and included some fish into her eating plan. I also recommended some natural digestive aids to balance her stomach acidity.

Her mood swings disappeared as soon as she included protein in all three meals. I put that down to the fact that she had blood sugar lows and highs (both extremes can create mood swings) which were now controlled. She still craved sweets, so I encouraged her to have more substantial snacks in between her meals such as:

- Rice cakes with guacamole
- Chickpea pâté with wheat free crackers
- Lentil rice salad
- Cashew butter on oat cakes

The balanced snacks cleared up the sweet cravings and slowed down her hair loss. Three weeks later her hair completely stopped falling out, by which time her stomach acid had improved too. Although Gillie was taking various thyroid supplements and eating pretty healthily she was not addressing her adrenal 'fight or flight' state, which had reduced her absorption and assimilation of food. For this reason she would have been on all these supplements for the rest of her life if she did not address the adrenal issue.

No more 'junk'

Gillie quit her ante natal group as it was creating more stress. The competitive environment was not conducive to her health. She cut down on so-called developmental activities for her baby, which helped him sleep better and Gillie and her partner got family counselling for new parents. Within 6 months she had addressed her 'stress' triggers, thereby supporting her adrenals and bounced back to the 'Gillie' her husband knew before the birth.

Joanne...single mum

Joanne was encouraged to put her son, Sam, on the Naked Truth lifestyle and to my delight the whole family started to follow the programme. She did not buy organic specififcally, but managed to include as much as she could. Cutting out sugar was easier than she thought as she discovered alternatives like sesame seed bars, nuts and seeds. Although some of the snacks had sugar in the form of honey or date syrup, my main goal was to remove all artificial colours and preservatives and balance Sam's blood sugar. This included eating fruits with some protein or fat rather than just fruit alone. This was actually cheaper and healthier than the so-called 'healthy snack bars'.

I advised that she ask her doctor to refer her son to a specialist for further investigations if necessary and not to go solely by the headmaster's observations.

When Joanne came back four weeks later, Sam had been seen by a specialist and had not been diagnosed with any condition and as far as the specialist could see he was 'absolutely fine'. Sam was doing much better at school, but there were the odd days where he would be slightly 'absent-minded, fidgety and sometimes disruptive' in class and it was always in the afternoons. I asked Joanne to keep a daily diary of what Sam was eating and also to ask him if he shared his lunch with his friends on any particular days. I had seen a similar case before. It turned out to be the E colours in the sweets that were being shared around at school lunch time. Sam was tested for sensitivities to various colourings and preservatives and he came up positive for one of the colourings that was present in this particular group of confectionery.

Joanne called a week later to say that his behaviour changed ONLY on the days he had a particular brand of sweets that were being 'kindly' shared around by his school friends. Once this was relayed to the headmaster these specific sweets were 'banned' and soon enough Sam was no longer having his 'behavioural' relapses.

Colourings and preservatives DO have a negative impact on children's learning capabilities and behaviour

Colourings and preservatives DO have a negative impact on children's learning capabilities and behaviour, as well as other toxic long-term effects that are not yet recognised. If you can eliminate such 'junk foods' from your children's school lunches, school grades may improve as well as their overall health!

Patricia ...The Bulimic

When Patricia came to see me, she had already returned her completed health profile questionnaire. From this I gathered that she had an eating disorder although she did not mention this in the questionnaire.

She had underlined the following symptoms: bloating, diarrhoea, muscle twitching, anxiety/depression, 'overweight', blood sugar lows (also known as hypoglycaemia), 'craving sweets', mood swings, breaking out in cold sweats, menstrual irregularities and cold extremities.

During the first session, she discussed her bulimia and pointed to exactly when it started. At the age of twenty one years she was raped by her 'boyfriend' and had only mentioned it to a close friend who encouraged her to seek therapy. It took six years before Patricia sought counselling. The very day she was raped she started to binge eat and from this it developed into bulimia. Even with over five years of therapy she had never been able to address her bulimia!

In the first session I did not want to address weight issues at all. It would have been like trying to 'fix' a dripping tap by wearing ear plugs. You block out the dripping sound but the tap is still dripping! She was in a state of 'desperation'. In her own words she said 'either I get free from this or the bulimia will kill me'. Patricia made the decision to 'get well'. Nutritionally she was very well read and like most other individuals with eating disorders feared fat. Her binges were at their worst when she was 'ravenous', so primarily she followed the Naked Truth lifestyle to balance her blood sugar levels especially during the day, so that by the evening she was not at the same 'extreme low blood sugar levels' as she was currently, which would reduce the intensity of a 'binge'. At the same time I also prescribed her a remedy for the emotional impact from the abuse that also encompassed bulimia as well as some of her 'suppressed anger' and referred her to a Cognitive Behavioural Therapist.

At the follow up session (within two weeks) her blood sugar levels were more stable and her mood swings had improved. Her bingeing had dropped from seven times a week to four. Her bowels were still not functioning as well as they were previous to her bulimia, so she was put on digestive supplements and also re-prescribed the same remedy for the emotional impact from the abuse.

By the time Patricia had had two sessions with the therapist and two sessions with me, she had not had a single binge in four weeks. Three months later she was completely free from bulimia.

Mary...the anti-ageing grand mother

Mary was born into a wealthy family and her parents travelled a lot due to her father's work. She went to boarding school at the age of eleven years and pretty much 'got on with it'. She loved studying and dived right into it. Mary excelled in every thing and did not expect anything less. In the first session she mentioned that she never wanted to be like her mother and independence was very important to her.

During Mary's University days she had been prescribed various medications as she had worked herself 'into the ground' and began to suffer from anxiety attacks. However, she graduated with a first class honours from Oxford and eventually went onto work just as hard at building her firm. She married in her mid-20s and had a daughter within two years. Her daughter went to boarding school, 'did well' professionally and married to have a daughter too.

Mary belonged to a variety of women's clubs and golf was one of her favourite past times. She spent a considerable amount of time and money on looking 'youthful'. When Mary came to see me it was mainly to keep the 'wrinkles' at bay. She was willing to make some changes to her eating habits, although she did not want it intruding too much into her lifestyle. It was important for me to address the fact that implementing the Naked Truth lifestyle was going to nourish her body physically but she also required emotional nourishment as she was deeply unhappy underneath her 'success'. I explained to Mary that the adrenals respond to emotional stress also which can hinder her health goals.

Mary's anti-ageing Naked Truth lifestyle involved removing several of the main toxins (the ageing factors) which were:

- alcohol
- synthetic hormones
- refined carbohydrates
- cosmetics that contained various chemicals such as parabens

And the introduction of nutrient and herbal support for her detox organs.

All the above toxins make the liver work twice as hard (to say the least). One of the reasons for ageing prematurely or unhealthily shall we say, is due to

The ageing process is very much an 'inside-out' as well as an 'outside-in' process

toxins flooding our bodies. When these toxins enter our bodies the detox organs such as the liver, kidneys, lungs, bowels and skin all have to work harder, doing longer shifts. This can age the detox organs. The ageing process is very much an 'inside-out' as well as an 'outside-in' process.

Anyone who is anti-ageing 'savvy' knows that:

- essential fatty acids (which are polyunsaturated fats that can not be made by the body but essential for the functioning of the body) are good for keeping the skin supple
- collagen is important for the elasticity of the skin
- vitamin A is a vital anti-oxidant in preventing wrinkles

These above supplements (be they in cosmetic form or nutrient form) are not of great benefit if the body is in 'fight or flight' mode.

As Mary followed the Naked Truth lifestyle not only did the texture of her skin improve but also her hair and she lost an extra few kilos as she came off the synthetic hormones which lightened the load on her liver and adrenals.

Over time, during sessions with Mary it came to light that she felt abandoned and unloved by her parents and that nothing was ever good enough for her father. She did her best at everything and excelled at everything she put her mind to, but it still did not get her father's approval. Mary felt that her mother was a 'victim' in life and she was not about to repeat it.

As Mary followed the Naked Truth lifestyle not only did the texture of her skin improve but also her hair and she lost an extra few kilos

When I asked why she was so 'busy' with her club associations she burst into floods of tears. Looking great on the outside does not 'fix' the inside and the adrenals will give it away in some form or another. So although I could help Mary dramatically on a physical level, her adrenals were still being stressed by her subconscious mind playing the same message again and again that her father did not really love her but loved what she achieved. The adrenals would register this message as subconscious stress as if she is in some sort of danger. This would then produce the famous stress hormone, cortisol which goes onto create all sorts of 'ageing' agents such as free radicals. Note here that adrenaline and cortisol in themselves can cause ageing due to their biochemical consequences.

Mary eventually went to see a psychotherapist to help address deeper issues of unhappiness.

The drive to age 'youthfully' is big business but when the drive is a detriment to overall health then the 'root' cause needs to be looked at.

The Gold Mind

Most of us have had or have some kind of what I call 'emotional toxicity' in our lives, be it through being in utero (unwanted child, lack of bonding, separation at birth, traumatic birth experience etc) childhood, (such as bullying, peer pressure, demanding parents) puberty (a shock in itself!), college, university, work, relationships to name just a few.

We have all heard that the mind is a powerful tool for success or failure in any area of life from losing weight through to building self-esteem. Most people grow up suppressing emotions and in specific cultures you can see this very clearly from any number of health issues such as eating disorders (usually amongst the more affluent) through to diabetes amongst the Indian community and tuberculosis in the migrating groups and so on. Unfortunately, we have become used to taking a pill for every ailment, to such a degree that some individuals are now on multiple medications all prescribed to combat the side effects of the previously prescribed medication.

We have to ask the question; 'Why is my body doing this?' I am a total believer not only in 'we are what we eat' BUT also 'we are what we think'.

It is not easy addressing the 'mind' especially when the mind has been pretty ingrained over years with stress, abuse, anger, jealousy, grief to name but a few, but the 'success' is worth every ounce of 'mental work'. The people that I mention had to address their thinking as well as eating habits, otherwise it just becomes another DIEt and six weeks later, we are back to square one.

The world of mind-body medicine has shown the link between an unhappy mind manifesting itself as a physical symptom. In very basic terms, we experience the world daily in two ways: one is through the conscious mind and the other through the subconscious mind. The conscious mind is the one we are fully aware of and think with daily. The subconscious mind is where all our memories, knowledge, emotions are stored and it is the most important aspect of the mind that needs to be addressed as far as health is concerned.

The science which is now being called psycho-neuro-immuno-endocrinology is the link between the mind, the nervous system, the immune system and the hormonal system

Science cannot prove how ALL this works, but the 'proof is in the pudding'. Candace Pert PhD discovered the exciting small molecules (called neuropeptides which are made from amino acids and come from our protein foods) which links the mind to the physical body. The science which is now being called psycho-neuro-immuno-endocrinology (known as PNIE for short) is sure to have a huge impact on the way medicine will be taught let alone practiced in our Western world in the future. In very simple terms,

PNIE is the link between the mind, the nervous system, the immune system and the hormonal system. It is unfathomable how Western medicine 'treats' the body as if it is made up of separately functioning parts.

There are many others who have done heavy duty studies on the mind-body connection who have helped their patients enormously. Dr. John Sarno, a mind-body medicine pioneer, beautifully illustrates and explains the link between the mind and back pain. This may make some of us feel a bit 'ridiculed' but this is more due to the belief that having some kind of an imbalance in the mind is seen as a 'weakness' and an embarrassment, when clearly this is not the case.

So if you are referred to an endocrinologist (hormone specialist) he or she should be asking when the symptoms started, what happened at that time in your life and whether you have any other symptoms such as an irritable bowel? What usually happens, however, is that we are sent off to different specialists for different conditions, such as the gastro-enterologist (gut specialist) for digestive issues or the endocrinologist for thyroid symptoms. Unfortunately, each one of these 'specialists' usually sees their particular speciality or 'compartment' walking in through the door rather than an individual. So when you are being referred to a specialist in most cases you will not be addressed as a 'whole' but as a dissected human being.

Science will probably have to make several U-turns and then some other turns in order to even start to understand the so-called 'mechanisms' behind the subconscious and the physical realm.

Most of us grow up repressing our emotions and the more these are repressed or ignored the more symptomatic the body becomes whether on an emotional level such as clinical

Mind body connection

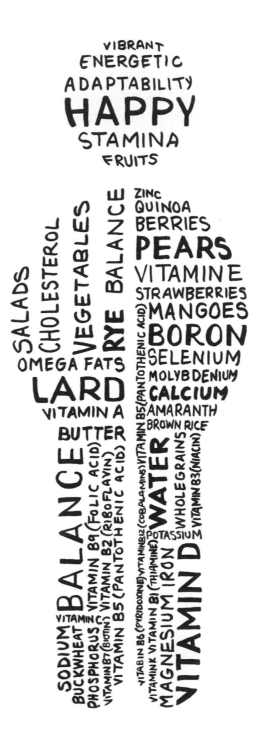

Mind body dis-connection

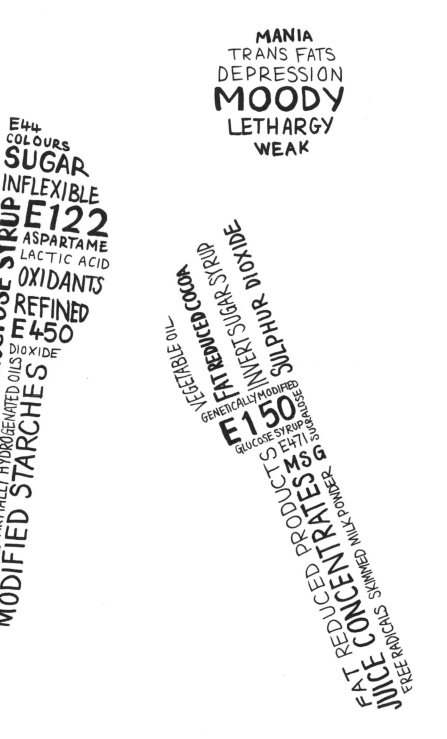

MANIA
TRANS FATS
DEPRESSION
MOODY
LETHARGY
WEAK

E44
COLOURS
SUGAR
INFLEXIBLE
E122
ASPARTAME
LACTIC ACID
OXIDANTS
REFINED
E450
DIOXIDE

GLUCOSE-FRUCTOSE SYRUP
TITANIUM **GLUCOSE**
E475
DEXTROSE E129 PARTIALLY HYDROGENATED OILS
MODIFIED STARCHES

VEGETABLE OIL
FAT REDUCED COCOA
INVERT SUGAR SYRUP
SULPHUR DIOXIDE
GENETICALLY MODIFIED
E150
GLUCOSE SYRUP E471 SUCRALOSE
MSG
PRODUCTS
FAT REDUCED
JUICE CONCENTRATES
FREE RADICALS SKIMMED MILK POWDER

depression or bulimia or on a physical level such as infertility, arthritis, back pain etc. When these physical symptoms arise, the body is crying out for help. It is trying to 'get your attention' and wants you to change something, be it your work environment, relationships, anger issues or anything else for that matter as well as your bad nutritional habits. Nowadays we numb that 'cry' with pills or denial but when we do that the symptoms only come back in another form and trying even harder to 'grab your attention' (in other words they tend to be more 'painful' and/or 'deeper'). The typical example being eczema (a skin condition) that turns into asthma (deeper lung imbalance). Doctors see it in practice and it is a well known 'phenomenon' but they are unable to explain it.

Take Kate, the girlfriend who is trying to lose a few pounds hoping one day she will marry her 'adrenalin high boyfriend'. Her desire to lose weight is coming from an unhealthy place, if she is trying to lose a few pounds to get back into last year's bikini that's different, but when she is doing this for someone else (denying her inner feelings), she is only 'harming herself'.

the more these are repressed or ignored the more symptomatic the body becomes whether on an emotional level such as clinical depression or bulimia or on a physical level such as infertility, arthritis, back pain

The 80:20 rule is pretty important here and by this I mean try and stick with eating healthily 80% of the time with 20% 'treat' time, but even as important is your emotional well being. What will you gain if you are eating healthily but are dissatisfied? As well as treating your body to the simplicity of the Naked Truth lifestyle give your mind a treat too!

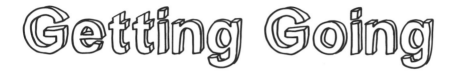

Getting Going

The basics

It is of vital importance that we address our food and follow the Naked Truth lifestyle before embarking on any of the recommended supplements. As mentioned previously there are no short cuts and the supplements are not short cuts in order to avoid eating well. The supplements recommended are supplementing the Naked Truth lifestyle not a substitute for the lifestyle.

I recommend a multivitamin and mineral to all my patients, whether they are already eating organic wholesome foods or not. This is because our farming methods and toxic environment is depleting the soil hence our foods of vital nutrients. Due to the free radical production that goes on daily especially due to stress and a toxic environment an anti-oxidant is implemented into the basic programme. Without a doubt some essential fatty acids known as omega oils are also recommended.

Supplement	Dose	Brand
*High Five (multivitamin and mineral formula) **OR** **Maximol Classic	One tablet a day with food Two tablespoons a day	Viridian Neways
**Astaxanthin and Blackcurrant (anti-oxidant)	One a day with a meal	Higher Nature
**Organic Flax seed oil (omega 3 oil with some omega 6 & 9)	One capsule a day with a meal	Higher Nature

* suitable for vegetarians
** suitable for vegetarians and vegans

Adrenal support

If you feel that you run on adrenaline or suffer from any of the 'itis' (which means inflammatory conditions such as colitis, arthritis, iritis, dermatitis, eczema etc) conditions or have allergies then I would recommend taking an adrenal support supplement. Also if your blood sugar has been yo-yoing over the past then it would also be of benefit to support your adrenals. I usually recommend a period of about 6 months at least to help stabilise them, but again if you know that you are going through a stressful time it is worth continuing to support them through this period whilst the stress is being addressed and not ignored. Add one of the adrenal support supplements overleaf to the basic supplement programme.

Supplement	Dose	Brand
Adreset (feeling run down)	One capsule three times a day with meals	Nutri Ltd.
Compose (feeling tired but internally 'wired')	One capsule three times a day with meals	Nutri Ltd.

** suitable for vegetarians and vegans

Digestive support

Enzymes

I recommend digestive enzymes for most people who start following to the Naked Truth lifestyle at the beginning for a minimum of 6 weeks. This is usually because the body has become used to eating less protein and/or fat, for this reason the clever body starts to reduce stomach acid levels accordingly and/or the pancreatic enzymes (usually both).

Firstly I would highly recommend trying out the stomach acid test, this is a quick and easy way to find out whether you have low stomach acid or not.

Stomach acid test

Take a teaspoon of organic apple cider vinegar and add it to a glass of water and drink. If you experience symptoms of slight 'burning' or indigestion then you have enough stomach acid...if you do not experience any symptoms then it seems that you have low stomach acid (again this is more common than not). For low stomach acid I would recommend either of the digestive enzyme supplements overleaf.

Supplement	Dose	Brand
High potency digestive aid (as well as enzymes contains ginger and peppermint)	One capsule with each meal	Viridian
Nutrigest (digestive enzymes with betaine HCl)	One tablet with each meal	Nutri Ltd.

** suitable for vegetarians and vegans.

Probiotics

These are 'good' bacteria in a pill and are absolutely vital for hormonal balance (especially in helping rid the body of toxic oestrogens) but also for boosting the immune system. Now if you are thinking well I am drinking plenty of the so-called yoghurts with lots of good bacteria, the sugar in these yoghurts is not really helping in colonising your gut with the so-called good bugs (the sugar could even be feeding the fungal folk!)...so the best way to implement this is to take a good probiotic.... and not to forget if you have been on antibiotics a probiotic is of utmost importance.

Supplement	Dose	Brand
**Bio-kult	Two capsules on an empty stomach	Protexin Healthcare

** suitable for vegetarians and vegans. The above probiotic can be stored at room temperature so great for travel too!

Liver and kidney support

For those:

- having stimulants regularly (yes this includes sugar, refined carbohydrates including 'fizzy' drinks, alcohol)
- who have been on prescription drugs or recreational drugs
- with adrenal stress

Supplement	Dose	Brand
**Liv drops and Kid drops	Twelve drops of each in a little water three times a day	Specialist Herbal Supplies

** suitable for vegetarians and vegans

So your supplement plan may look like this:

Supplement	Dose	Brand
High five	One tablet a day with food	Viridian
Compose	One capsule three times a day with meals	Nutri Ltd.
Astaxanthin and Blackcurrant	One a day with a meal	Higher Nature
Bio-kult	Two capsules on an empty stomach	Protexin
Liv and Kid drops	Twelve drops of each in a little water three times a day	Specialist Herbal Supplies
Organic Flax seed oil (omega 3 oil with some omega 6 & 9)	One capsule two times a day with meals	Higher Nature

Protein shakes

To date the easiest and efficient way that I have found to 'heal' a 'leaky' gut is by using a well balanced protein powder, ideally one that you are not 'intolerant' to. There are various protein powders on the market, my firm favourite is the Vianesse which is both dairy and gluten free but also tastes great, which helps! However there are various others, which I also mention and you can take your pick.

I generally recommend a protein 'shake' once a day for 6 weeks but some people continue with these 'shakes' as they find them convenient as well as healthy especially for breakfast or mid afternoon snack.

To maintain the blood sugar balance stick with the whole carbohydrate:protein:fat combination, I would not suggest adding fruit juice to the powder.

Protein powder	Dose	Brand
Body Shape (lactalbumin based)	Once a day	Vianesse
BioPure Protein (whey based)	Once a day	Nutri Ltd.
Energy Breakfast Shape (seed based with rice protein and quinoa)	Once a day	Higher Nature

* suitable for vegetarians
** suitable for vegetarians and vegans

Recipe

Take 2-3 scoops of the powder and add 200ml of milk (for example rice milk, oat milk, almond or quinoa milk, (personally I would not recommend dairy milk). Mix in a blender or in a shaker. You can add some fruit (apple/pear/banana/berries etc) you can also add vanilla essence for additional flavour or ground cinnamon. Two tablespoons of nut butter and some flax seeds also known as linseeds approx. two tablespoons. Blend and drink.

Alternatively, you can put together your own ingredients to the protein powder just ensure that you add carbohydrate and fat to the powder. This also creates a low glycaemic load shake (prevents the blood sugar surge, keeps adrenals 'happy'). Protein shakes are gentler on the digestive system and this recipe can provide a nutrient dense meal/snack. If you would like to flavour your shake you may want try any of the 'tips' below or use your own creative ideas;

i. Chocolate; I would recommend adding good quality organic cocoa powder (check it has no sugar in the ingredients label)

ii. Vanilla; can add a few drops or so (according to your taste) of vanilla essence with or without a pinch of ground cinnamon

iii. Coconut; you can add a tablespoon of coconut oil as the fat

The supplements can be ordered from www.khushmark.com and the Vianesse protein powder can be ordered from www.mandimart.co.uk

Nutritionise me in a few minutes

- Try to drink **water** throughout the day, at least enough to ensure that your urine is clear and not yellow which usually means **at least** 1.0 litre of water a day. I would not recommend drinking tap water unless it is filtered by good quality water filters such as the reverse osmosis filters (our tap water is becoming more and more polluted with not only toxic metals but synthetic pharmaceutical bi-products) or have the bottled variety but it is worth investing in a reverse osmosis water filter long-term

- Eat **organic food** as much as possible

- **Every meal** should include a carbohydrate, a protein and fat. This is important in maintaining the body's blood sugar levels preventing the adrenals from having to come in and work which utilises the body's vital energy that would otherwise be used to heal and repair the body

- Have 3 meals a day with snacks in between as necessary...do not go longer than 4 **hours without food**, this sets you up for the blood sugar 'yo-yo' effect all day long, stressing the adrenals, which robs the body of energy

- **Every snack** should include a carbohydrate with either a protein OR fat. Choose healthy options such as a piece of fruit with some nuts or seeds, or fruit with yoghurt or carrots/cucumber with houmous or guacamole. Try not to eat fruit (a carbohydrate) on its own (or any other form of sugar), it can create a blood sugar imbalance which can cause stress on the adrenals preventing optimal health

- **Carbohydrates** include: **vegetables, salads, wholegrains** (brown rice, amaranth, quinoa, buckwheat etc), potatoes, pasta and fruit. Those in bold are ideal. Have fruit with fat (such as nuts and seeds) or any protein (such as yoghurt) but not on their own. It is very important to eat regularly in order to maintain healthy blood sugar levels. I would not recommend dried fruit as an alternative to fresh fruit as it is pretty concentrated in fruit sugar

- **Proteins** include: meat, fish, lentils and pulses, dairy products and fermented soya products. Have protein at **every** meal

- **Fats** include: butter, clarified butter/ghee, olive oil, nuts and their oils. Include fat with **EVERY** main meal

- Avoid **ALL** hydrogenated fats (also known as trans fats/ partially hydrogenated fats) **as much as possible**. They are usually found in ready made meals and snacks such as **crisps, chocolate bars, biscuits, mayonnaise** and also in most margarine. Such fats have been shown to cause various biological imbalances in the body. Foods that contain such fats are now being labelled in the USA with a health warning

- Heating vegetable or seed oils can create free radicals which are harmful to general well-being, so do not cook with these oils. Cook with palm oil, butter, coconut oil or clarified butter (this is in no particular order, just whatever you prefer). GOOD fat is not bad for you

- Have at least a plate full of steamed vegetables every day or a salad as part of your main meal

- Avoid **ALL** stimulants as much as possible (such as sugar, chocolate, caffeine, pastries, white flour products in general) as they are known to play havoc with blood sugar regulation and therefore health

- If interested there is an alternative to sugar that does not affect the pancreas/adrenal balance called xylitol. Xylitol does not have any effects on insulin levels and also does not contain or produce toxic bi-products in the body. You can use this for baking, cooking, adding to hot drinks etc. It is available in some food stores such as Sainsbury's in the 'well being section'

- The various alternatives to dairy milk that you may want to try are: organic oat milk, almond milk or quinoa milk. Remember that these milk options do not have much protein so you will want an additional protein source(s) such as a good protein powder or with a boiled egg or with some fat like some nut butter mixed into the milk. CURRENTLY I do not believe that soya milk is a healthy alternative to dairy milk, I feel more research needs to be done on soya in its varying forms

- Try and eat seeds daily (pumpkin, sesame and flax) as not only are they rich in various minerals but they also contain essential fats. I would encourage you to take between 1-2 tablespoons of ground (must be ground to obtain the full benefits) flax seeds a day. You can sprinkle this on any warm or cold foods (not hot) for example a salad or in a protein shake. However, you will need to grind the flax seeds (grind enough for 4 days and store the ground powder in a glass air-tight container in the fridge). **Do not store ground flax seeds that have been exposed to air longer than 5 days** as they become rancid. Ideally grind fresh seeds every 4-5 days. The ground flax seeds are great for regulating bowel movement but also for detoxification purposes. The advantage of having flax seeds over flax oil is that the seeds contain the fibre (the oil does not). All you need is a small electric pepper/coffee grinder for grinding the seeds (not used for anything else, so avoiding 'flavour contamination')

- It is important that meals are varied and try to eat raw fruits and vegetables daily as part of snacks and/or meals

- Try and have some **virgin** coconut oil (about a teaspoon daily). You can add it to a protein shake if desired or cook with the oil. Coconut oil is also known to boost the thyroid and hence the metabolism and has many other healing properties

- Avoid using microwaves to heat or cook food. Microwaves deplete ALL foods of vital energy

- Use the Himalayan salt or the Celtic sea salt also known as the French 'Gros Sel de Guerande' salt as it contains various minerals and is not based on sodium chloride. It is important that we have this unrefined salt daily. We should not be avoiding healthy wholesome salt BUT avoiding regular refined table salt.

Naked Truth Lifestyle: Weekly Menu Plan

Non vegetarian meal plan

Day	Breakfast	Lunch	Snack	Dinner
one	Natural yoghurt with muesli & fruit	Rocket prawn & avocado salad Yoghurt	A piece of fruit with a nut mix	Omelette with grilled vegetables & potatoes fried in butter
two	Porridge oats with ground almonds & a protein shake	Chicken rye bread sandwich with a salad on the side Fruit	Almond butter on chopped banana	Salmon with roasted vegetables & wild rice with cashews
three	Scrambled eggs with rye bread toast & grilled tomatoes	Chilli con carne & brown rice with side salad	Fruit salad with yoghurt	Roast lamb with roast potatoes & greens
four	Protein powder shake with berries, quinoa milk & macadamia nut butter	Herb crusted lamb chops with garlic butter & sautéed vegetables and fruit salad	Cottage cheese with pineapple	Salad for starter & chicken curry with brown basmati rice

Non vegetarian meal plan cont...

Day	Breakfast	Lunch	Snack	Dinner
five	Barley & oat porridge with banana, nuts & seeds with almond milk sprinkling of protein powder	Poached salmon with new potatoes & cucumber salad	Seed bar with a fruit	Lamb moussaka with a salad piece of organic dark chocolate
six	Egg with sausages & grilled tomatoes and mushrooms	Tuna salad Yoghurt	Apple with some cheese	Thai take out ice cream
seven	Spinach omelette with grilled tomatoes & potatoes fried in butter	Salad nicoise with yoghurt smoothie	Chick pea pate with cucumber sticks	Steak with steamed vegetables Fruit salad

More non vegetarian meal plans can be found at www.khushmark.com

Vegetarian meal plan

Day	Breakfast	Lunch	Snack	Dinner
one	Natural yoghurt with muesli & fruit	Avocado & mozzarella green herb salad yoghurt	Fruit & nut mix	Spinach omelette with grilled vegetables and potatoes fried in butter
two	Porridge oats with ground almonds & a protein shake	Cheese rye bread sandwich with a salad on the side Fruit	Almond butter on chopped banana	Lentil moussaka Fruit salad
three	Scrambled eggs with rye bread toast & grilled tomatoes	Mediterranean style bean salad with rye crackers	Fruit salad with yoghurt	Rocket salad and lentil stew with barley
four	Protein powder with berries, quinoa milk & macadamia nut butter	Chickpea salad seed bar	Cottage cheese with spelt crackers	Salad for starter & Mixed bean curry with brown basmati rice
five	Greek yoghurt chocolate shake with vanilla essence	Tofu with stir fried vegetables	Seed bar with a fruit	Asparagus with poached egg & tarragon butter Nuts & seeds

Vegetarian meal plan cont...

Day	Breakfast	Lunch	Snack	Dinner
six	Cottage cheese with pineapple & sprinkled seeds	Black bean chilli & yoghurt with fruit salad	Spicy red lentil pate with celery	Thai take out ice cream
seven	Herb omelette with mustard mushrooms	Bean burger with rye bread & green salad Yoghurt fruit smoothie	Chick pea pate with cucumber sticks	Warm lentil broccoli salad piece of organic dark chocolate

More vegetarian meal plans can be found at www.khushmark.com

Glossary

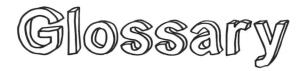

Adrenal fatigue: adrenal glands that have reduced ability to respond to stress efficiently.

Adrenal glands: two glands that sit on top of the kidneys, primary response is to deal with stress of any kind.

Amino acids: the building blocks of proteins as well as intermediates in metabolism.

Antioxidants: compounds that prevent or delay undesirable oxidation.

Arteries: blood vessels that carry blood away from the heart

Arteriosclerosis: a thickening of the blood vessel walls and loss of elasticity in the small and medium sized arteries.

Atherosclerotic plaque: a deposit of fat and other substances that accumulate in the lining of the arterial wall.

Carbohydrates: a food group that provides the body with energy. Like a fuel in an engine they 'burn' in the presence of oxygen providing four calories per gram.

Cholesterol: a type of fat made by the body and also found in some foods. This fat is important in the synthesis of various sex hormones, vitamin D and stress hormone cortisol.

Cold pressed: description given to a food oil that has been extracted from a seed or grain without the use of high temperatures or solvents.

Cortisol: stress hormone produced by the adrenals and made from cholesterol.

Enzymes: biochemical catalysts.

Fats: a food group that provides the most concentrated form of energy provides nine calories per gram. Fats can be divided into saturated in that they are solids and unsaturated fats are oils.

Glycaemic Index: an index ranking the effects of various foods on blood glucose levels.

Hydrogenated fats: liquid oils that have been turned into hard fats by hydrogenation.

Hydrogenation: process whereby liquid oil is reacted under pressure with hydrogen gas at 250 - 400°F for several hours in the presence of a catalyst such as nickel or platinum. This artificial process converts liquid fats into solids such as margarine.

Inflammation: a localised immune response triggered by injury or damaged tissues which is protective to the body allowing the body to deal with the injury as well triggering the healing process.

Pancreas: a gland in the body responsible for digestion as well as blood sugar control through it's production of insulin

Partially hydrogenated fats: fats that are incompletely hydrogenated also known as trans fat. These are worse than totally hydrogenated fats.

pH: the concentration of hydrogen ions. Low pH also known as acidic pH corresponds to high concentration of hydrogen ions. High pH also known as alkaline pH corresponds to low concentration of hydrogen ions.

Physiological: appropriate to an organism's healthy or normal functioning.

Proteins: a food group that consists of amino acids and has numerous functions including growth, immunity, hormones, enzymes. Provides four calories per gram. It is the most plentiful substance in the body after water.

Refined carbohydrates: whole grains that have been stripped of important nutrients such a B vitamins by removing the bran and the germ of the grain. These include anything made from flour, milled corn or white rice.

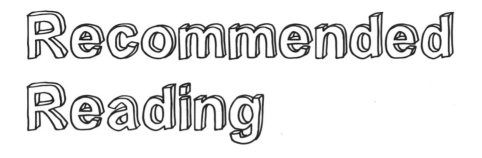

Recommended Reading

Batmanghelidj F. Your Body's Many Cries for Water: You Are Not Sick, You Are Thirsty. 1997. Global Health Solutions Inc.

Gittleman AL. Get the Sugar Out: 501 Simple Ways to Cut the Sugar Out of Any Diet. 1996. Three Rivers Press.

Cousins N. Anatomy of an Illness as Perceived by the Patient. 1979. W.W. Norton and Company Ltd.

Enig MG. Know Your Fats: The Complete Primer for Understanding The Nutrition of Fats, Oils and Cholesterol. 2000. Bethesda Press

Gershon M. The Second Brain: The Scientific Basis of Gut Instinct and a Groundbreaking New Understanding of Nervous Disorders of the Stomach and Intestines. 1998. Harper Collins

Pert C. Molecules of Emotion: The Science Behind Mind Body Medicine. 1999. Touchstone

Ravnskov U. The Cholesterol Myths. Exposing the Fallacy that Saturated Fat and Cholesterol Cause Heart Disease. 2000. New Trends Publishing

Sapolsky R. Why Zebras Don't Get Ulcers. 2004. Saint Martin's Press

Sarno JE. The Divided Mind: The Epidemic of Mindbody Disorders. 2006. Harper Collins.

Taubes G. The Diet Delusion: Challenging the Conventional Wisdom on Diet, Weight Loss and Disease. 2008. Vermilion

Weston A Price. Nutrition and Physical Degeneration. 1939. New Trends Publishing

Wolcott W. The Metabolic Typing Diet. 2000. Doubleday

Final Thoughts

I hope you have found that healthy living is not complicated but that it is a simple and effective lifestyle.

To great health!

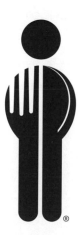

www.khushmark.com

About the author

Khush Mark PhD, is a consultant and lecturer in nutrition. She ran a successful practice in New York before moving back to the UK, where she has been running a practice in Harley Street, London since 2002. Her educational background includes a BSc in Pharmacology, MSc in Toxicology and Pathology, a PhD in cancer from Kings College, London, and an MSc in Human Nutrition which allows her to connect her theoretical knowledge to her clinical practice. Her work has been published in various health magazines, national as well as international newspapers.

Khush's motto 'you are what you think as well as what you eat', stems from her clinical observations in practice, which has led her to implement mind-body medicine into her practice.

Khush lives with her husband and two sons, in Kingston-Upon-Thames, Surrey. www.khushmark.com